# THE BIG FAT
## ACTIVITY BOOK
### FOR PREGNANT PEOPLE

*For Bonnie and Linda, who had big fat pregnancies with us*

**tarcher**perigee

An imprint of Penguin Random House LLC
375 Hudson Street
New York, New York 10014

Copyright © 2017 by Jordan Reid and Erin Williams

TarcherPerigee with tp colophon is a registered trademark of Penguin Random House LLC.

Most TarcherPerigee books are available at special quantity discounts for bulk purchase for sales promotions, premiums, fund-raising, and educational needs. Special books or book excerpts also can be created to fit specific needs. For details, write: SpecialMarkets@penguinrandomhouse.com.

LIBRARY OF CONGRESS CATALOGING-IN-PUBLICATION DATA has been applied for.

ISBN 9780735213685 (paperback)
ISBN 9780735213692 (eBook)

Printed in the United States of America
10   9   8   7

Neither the publisher nor the author is engaged in rendering professional advice or services to the individual reader. The ideas, procedures, and suggestions contained in this book are not intended as a substitute for consulting with your physician. All matters regarding your health require medical supervision. Neither the author nor the publisher shall be liable or responsible for any loss or damage allegedly arising from any information or suggestion in this book.

Book design by Erin Williams

# THE BIG FAT
# ACTIVITY BOOK
## FOR PREGNANT PEOPLE

A TARCHERPERIGEE BOOK

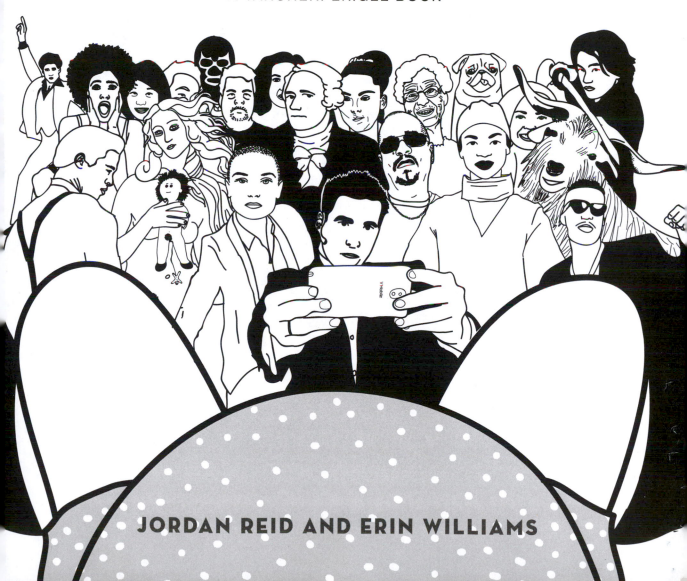

JORDAN REID AND ERIN WILLIAMS

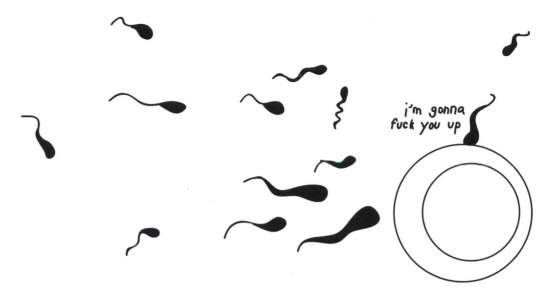

i'm gonna fuck you up

# DEAR PREGNANT PERSON,

Pregnancy can be magical. You get to spend nine months with the person who will be your very best friend in the world growing inside you, except they're not here yet, so instead of going to Build-A-Bear on Saturday (again and again and again), you can do things like nothing, or Netflix.

Pregnancy can also be its own special kind of hell. Your feet turn into twin Goodyear Blimps. Parts of your body hurt that you didn't even know existed. Everyone you encounter on the street will try to touch you and then assert their opinion about what you're doing wrong, which is everything. And around Month 8, you stop being able to get out of bed to use the bathroom without an assistant and/or bulldozer—and let us tell you, being physically rolled in the direction of the toilet like a sweaty whale (complete with considerable huffing and puffing on the part of the person with whom you are allegedly having a deeply romantic love affair) is both as elegant as it sounds and absolutely spectacular for the ol' self-esteem.

And beyond that, you likely have quite a lot on your mind. In addition to the usual money/house/relationship stresses, you now must add "the care and cultivation of a human life" to your list of responsibilities. Are you taking the right vitamins? Was your doctor joking when she asked if you're exercising? Was that the sound of maternity pants ripping? Why won't the baby stop kicking you in the ribs? And OH MY GOD THE BABY HASN'T KICKED IN FOURTEEN MINUTES DO I NEED TO START COUNTING?

The answer to all of the above is: You are fine. In fact, you are amazing.

You're building a person from scratch! And you're doing a great job. (And yes, your doctor was joking when she told you to exercise; what she actually meant was "eat pizza while lying down.") No matter what you're worrying about, you are not alone. We all have these fears—almost constantly—for nine (or ten!) months.

We're here to tell you that it's okay. And you look spectacular today, did we mention that? Your ankles look very slender. You can barely see the BBQ sauce on your blouse.

We're also here to distract you. Inside this book you'll find tons and tons of spirit-lifting activities, games, and stories to remind you that you've got this. (And also to tell you to remember that when it comes to pregnancy, step away from The Google, because what Google does to pregnant people is it makes them panic. Try an activity or two instead; they're way more fun than panicking.)

Love,
Jordan and Erin

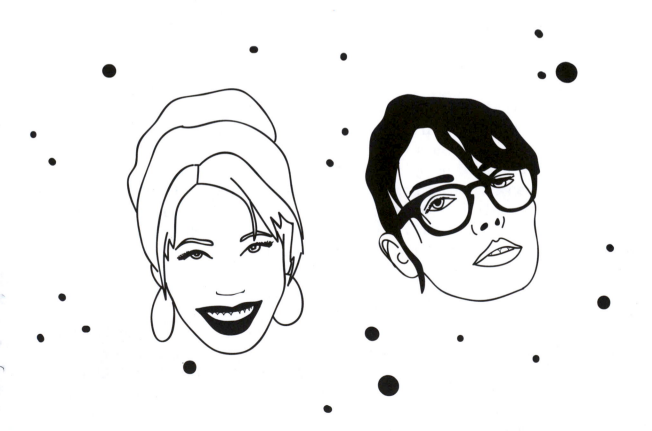

# HOW TO USE THIS BOOK

1. Pick it up whenever the mood hits: in the morning, to distract you from your blinding desire for a caffeine IV drip; during your lunch break (we strongly recommend grilled cheese; see page 17); late at night, when the hippopotamus-size pillow propping up your stomach just isn't doing the trick and you can't sleep.

2. The book is loosely divided by trimester, but don't worry about reading it cover to cover: The point is to chill you out, so do an activity, skip ahead to an essay, flip back to a journal entry, color in a picture—whatever you want. Write notes in the margins. Doodle. You have approximately eighteen years ahead of you, during which you will be highly unlikely to hear the words "Oh, do whatever you want!," so you might as well take advantage now.

3. If you're so inclined, take a picture of your creations and tag us on Instagram @bigactivitybook—we want to see (and share) your genius!

# OH SHIT

# I'M PREGNANT

## THE FIRST TRIMESTER

# ALL ABOUT ME

Hello. My name is _____, I am pregnant, and this is my book.

I am _____ years old.

I am:
- a) Single
- b) In a relationship
- c) Married
- d) Let's not discuss

I found out I was pregnant when:
- a) I peed on a stick
- b) My boobs suddenly became porn star–ish
- c) I woke up one morning and discovered that I had transformed into the emotional equivalent of a tsunami
- d) Other _____

I'm planning to give birth:
- a) At a hospital, duh
- b) In a bathtub
- c) In my bed, surrounded by candles and the soothing strains of Enya
- d) Anywhere but in my car, please
- e) Other _____

What I'm most excited about for this pregnancy is:
- a) The boobs
- b) My new shape
- c) Eating my weight in Ritz Crackers
- d) Experiencing the miracle of childbirth
- e) Other _____

What I'm least excited about for this pregnancy is:
- a) The boobs
- b) My new shape
- c) The fact that I will want to eat All The Things
- d) Experiencing the miracle of childbirth
- e) Other _____

I'm having:
- a) A boy
- b) A girl
- c) A human being
- d) More than one of the above, and how I feel about this is _____

I do/don't have a name picked out yet. (It's _____, and my mother/best friend/sister is going to love/hate it.)

When I think about the fact that I am about to have a baby, I feel:
- a) Excited
- b) Terrified
- c) Overwhelmed
- d) Confused
- e) Like I want to cry in a happy way
- f) Like I want to cry in a not-happy way
- g) Like I need a sandwich

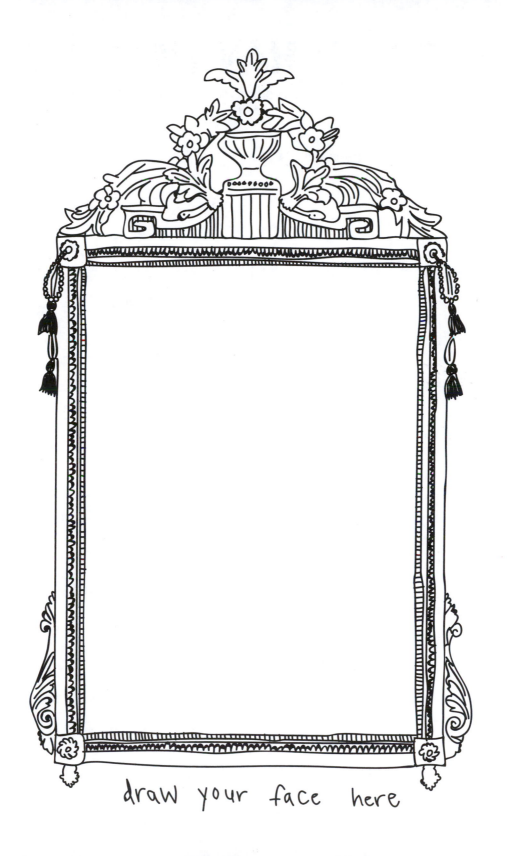

draw your face here

# I'M TOTALLY HAVING A BABY!

*Hand this page over to a partner, who will prompt you for each blank, then read your epic creation out loud.*

Here is how I found out I was pregnant:

It was a(n) _____, _____ _____. I
               adjective           adjective        day of the week

woke up at _____ and headed into the _____, bringing my
        time of day                  room

_____ along with me. I sat down on the _____ and started
   object                      piece of furniture

to _____. Slowly, the _____ turned _____!
   verb           same object        color

"_____!" I said.
  exclamation

I ran into the _____ and woke up _____. "Honey,"
         room              person

I said, "I'm so _____ I could _____. We're having a
        adjective          verb

_____!"
  noun

"_____!" said _____.
   exclamation        person

The first thing we did was head to _____ to eat some
               restaurant

_____ and drink some _____. Then we went home,
  food           drink

lay down on the _____, and _____. It was so
     piece of furniture    gesture of affection, past tense

_____. After some discussion, we decided that we're going to put your crib
 adjective

in the _____, and paint the walls with pictures of _____.
   room                    noun, plural

Over your bed, I'm thinking we'll hang a(n) _____. It's going to be SO
                        noun

_____.
 adjective

They tell me that right now you're the size of a _____, but I think I'll
                         vegetable

just call you my little _____.
         baked good

# THINGS YOU CAN DO NOW THAT YOU'RE PREGNANT

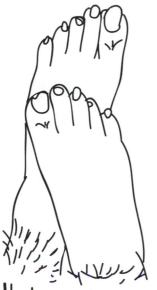

forget that you have toenails

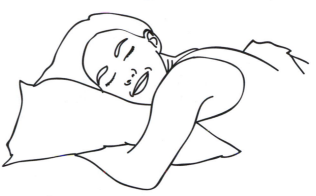

demand extra sleep "for the baby"

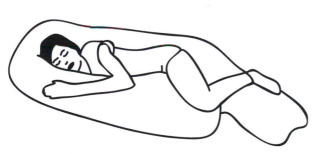

replace your partner with a $200 pillow

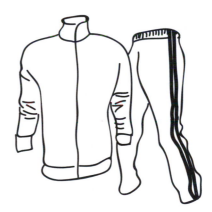

wear pajamas ("athleisure suits") to the office

# Quiz

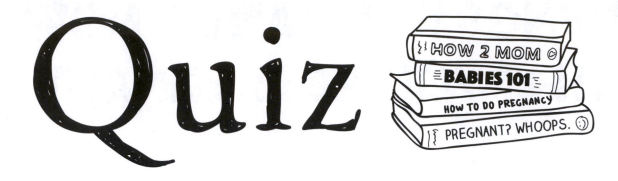

# WHAT'S YOUR BASE KNOWLEDGE LEVEL?

When you're newly pregnant, you get to spend a few weeks in a magical, joyful state in which you are not yet retaining a virtual ocean of water and are also not being bombarded with information from everyone from the lady on line behind you at CVS to your mother-in-law's geriatric second cousin Alice.

You may know a lot. You may know a little. It doesn't really matter either way, because by the time you get to the finish line, you will know it ALL (or at least you'll know what you need to know, which is about one one-thousandth of what you'll end up knowing).

*Find out what you know right this very second.*

1. What is "vernix"?
    a) Plural for "vulva" (as an example, your gynecologist might say, "Ay, the vernix I've seen in my day!")
    b) The girl version of a taint
    c) Baby cheese
    d) The emotion you feel toward your dog when he pees on the corner of the bed

2. Which of these can you not do now that you're pregnant?
    a) Shave your bikini line
    b) Have sex
    c) Pick stuff up
    d) Be emotionally stable

3. Speaking of sex, what's the best position when pregnant?
    a) Missionary style
    b) Doggy style
    c) That thing where you both lay on your side that never actually works
    d) The depth of my not-caring is infinite

4. Which of these substances are you allowed to ingest during pregnancy?
   a) Heroin
   b) Aspirin
   c) Tuna sashimi
   d) A nice gooey brie

5. What is the "afterbirth"?
   a) The umbilical cord
   b) The placenta
   c) The excess fluid that's still in your body for a couple of weeks after you have the baby
   d) The part where someone brings you wine

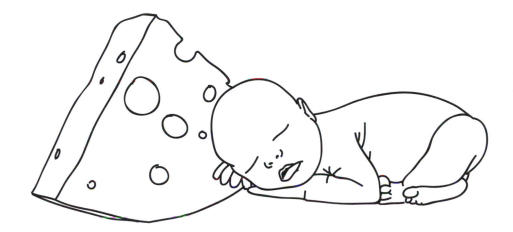

# answers

1. (c) It's baby cheese (that's a scientific term, in case you were wondering), and your child will be covered with it when he or she emerges from your body. It's as attractive as it sounds.

2. You can still do all these things. But you get to use pregnancy as an excuse to not do them.

3. Whatever sexual position is comfortable for you is A-OK, even if said position is "GET OFF." You're making life. You do what you want, girlfriend.

4. You can't have any of these. Isn't that annoying?

5. Technically the afterbirth is (b), the placenta, but it should also refer to (d), the part where someone realizes that you have been deprived of shiraz for nine entire months and brings it to you in a goddamn urine cup if they have to.

# WHEN YOU DOWNLOAD THAT APP THAT TELLS YOU WHAT FRUIT YOUR BABY IS AND SKIP AHEAD AND SEE "WATERMELON" AND POSSIBLY COLLAPSE

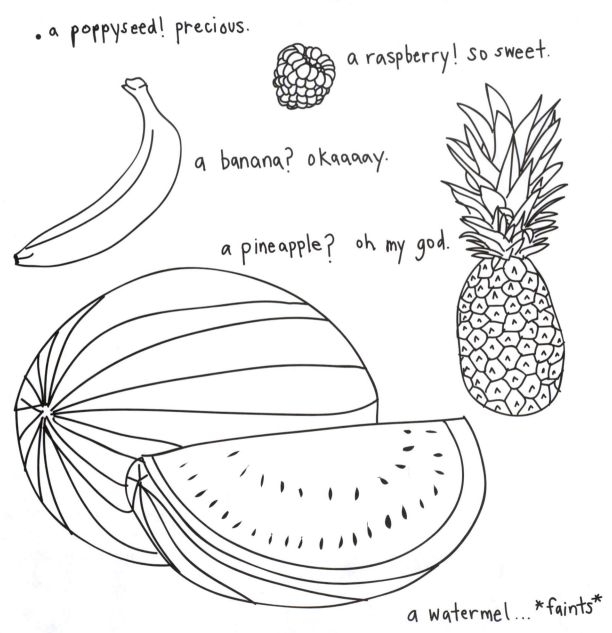

. a poppyseed! precious.

a raspberry! so sweet.

a banana? okaaaay.

a pineapple? oh my god.

a watermel...*faints*

# DRAW YOUR FUTURE

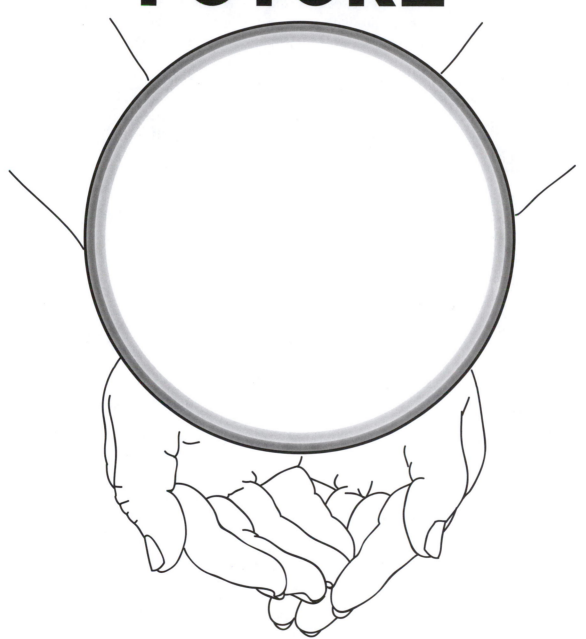

# SORRY, NOPE

*Locate the hidden words describing things that may have previously been an intimate part of your existence but are presently off limits unless you want someone to yell at you. (Except for missionary-style sex. You can technically do that . . . we think . . . but it sounds really uncomfortable. Also please be aware that we obviously partook in some of these things during our own pregnancies because sometimes a good ham sandwich is non-optional.)*

BODY SHOTS

BOTTLE OF WINE

CAT LITTER

CIGARETTE

COOKIE DOUGH

DRUGS

ESPRESSO

GOOD CHEESE

HAM SANDWICH

HOT BATH

HOT DOG

LISTERIA

MARTINI

MISSIONARY STYLE SEX

PATE

RAW EGGS

SUSHI

TEQUILA

TRAMPOLINE

TUNA FISH

WATER SKIING

XRAY

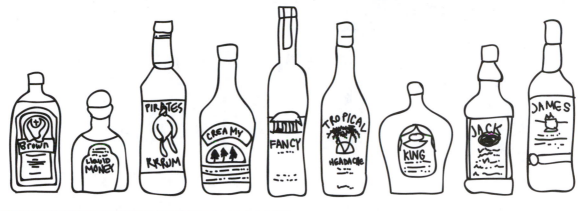

```
T H F R T S Q J C Y B K Y Q Y V X H L E T N M D D V O A E A
A L S Z A U R A A H D O Y S A O U E K R H O A K O D N O N M I
D N D T I C W T A T G G A D O R H G U O D E I K O O C I S U R
H S T V F L A E A Q X D T U Y X X E Z L I U L E W G L G R E E
F C G A I A B G O S E R P S E C A F K M I X Q O X K V V T S T
A U I T V T N J G Z M C V S R Q H P V R V U J Z A P O N G N S I
A F T W O G N N U D S Q V E V N P O H R V Q L M P B X Y N I L L
K E M H D S N E T T B G V H I C S T P O G A X G H F W F X L R P
R U I V H P N T R N L I Y T C K S S R Z N S N C L J L Y S R W H
S T S S V Z A A P Z A H K Y C R W X B T T G S H R W P S O L A R
C N S S P Q K S P Z R Y B G V U O B E U Z O G H E S Q P P S W S
Y K I J P E R O I M L R J I C Z T D O E Q T L W U P K F M L Z U
Q O V G Q B S R A G T G N T R V D A D G D G P R T E W I O A N N
E P N R D A T Y X L P E H X I L N Y G T O I P G W N N D O J I O T
O B A A D V R I Y S E J I E O B U I G W I Q A K H K W L S L U T
C J O R Q A T K L D G O O D C H E E S E W O L X J Z V F O A L X U
I R Y S P Z B M Y S L U F Z Z U P H X M G G Q Y G Q R K D T X J E
G W S B C O B B R W H U B G D Q M A R R I N I T S V E S T L C I C
A W T J I E T K I H E K R Y I W T Q R Y S O P E C R S J L L L E C
R W Y O C M E N X N V G P O K I X A P X Y F O Q W T W Q F H P H C
E X L Z M T E Q M C U N I E C W B N O G W K L U H X M Z T T I E O
T C E Q E J R X T U M I S X T G M T I W C T W I W M Q H V E B X Q
T F S L Q D K M B L S I V C G Z I D R A J T V L Y M R S V P C X O
E P E M A A P T K H N K Y J E Y S D X X Q I T A M W U E H O K K E
T N X G T G Y T M R E S W U S D S C O M H N G O Q G S O W I L O K
B T E D L B A F L N R J Z W X Q Q X Q G N G O Q G S O W I L O K
T K J P U D X G L O R E Z K L B X J K R S K D C T N M I T H E O K
B C Z R A N D Z Z G L T U K M P E A M B T H Z D L T H O I E K
N E N V R B L M N X S A D K H A C D N E M Q E D Y L M E I B W
V Y I H S U S E S N D W W X B F R N I K L H C A X I C X B W
```

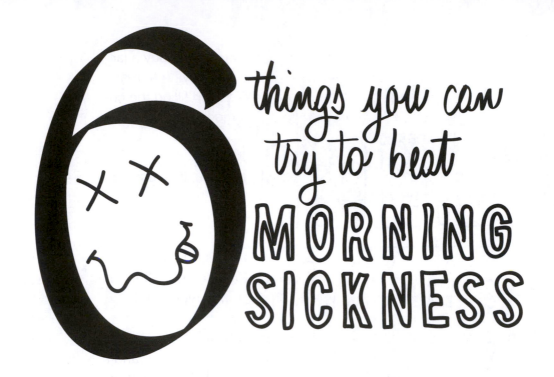

# 6 things you can try to beat MORNING SICKNESS

Have you ever been on a small boat in choppy waters with a bad hangover and an uncle who makes mouth sounds? Hello, first trimester. (For some people. For those of you who sail through all blissful and vomitless, congratulations; you are officially a Pregnancy Miracle.)

Everyone you know (and everyone on the Internet) will be more than happy to hand over lots of folksy advice on how to combat morning sickness. These remedies will probably not work, but what the hell: They're worth a shot.

Said advice may include:

**1. Fancy Motion Sickness Bracelets**
You can buy these online for $19. If you wear one, everyone will know you're pregnant because (a) you're not on a boat, and (b) these are not fashionable accessories. Unless you regularly wear a sweatband on each wrist to complement your power suit, consider yourself outed.

**2. Aromatherapy**
Some people swear by the mind-and-body-altering power of smells and will try to convince you to purchase a small vial of peppermint oil to whip out when you're feeling sick. If this works for you, please email us with the subject line "I Was Cured by Smells" and tell us about your experience.

### 3. Fennel Seeds

Because your first trimester isn't punishing enough, you should buy a jar of tiny seeds seasoned with Essence of Armpit and chew on them while trying to restrain yourself from puking. Bonus: Enjoy the sensation of licorice-flavored sand filling the crevices between your teeth. This remedy could only have been invented by men.

### 4. Sour Candy

Regardless of whether or not this "cure" is actually effective, it gives you an excuse to eat Sour Patch Kids by the pound, so that's good.

### 5. Grilled Cheese

Many women try to stave off the effects of morning sickness by ensuring that they never get too hungry, and a grilled cheese alongside your morning cup of coffee isn't the worst way to start your day. (Saltines help, too, but cheesy bread is way more fun.)

### 6. Simultaneous Back Massage and Chocolate Cake

Okay, we made this one up. But pregnancy is a great excuse to demand a lot of favors from your partner and/or anyone in your immediate vicinity, and we suggest you take advantage of that. With massages. And cake.

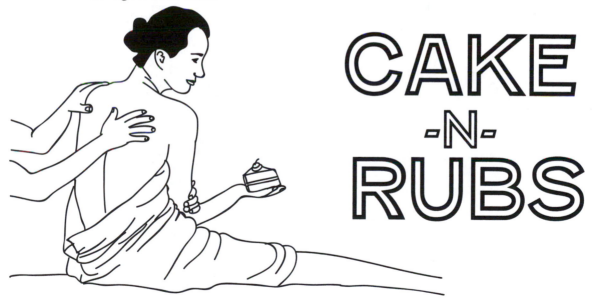

P.S. There are plenty of safe and effective medicines for morning sickness out there. If you're all full up on fennel seeds, go have a chat with your doctor.

# SMELLS THAT MAKE YOU WANT TO HURL

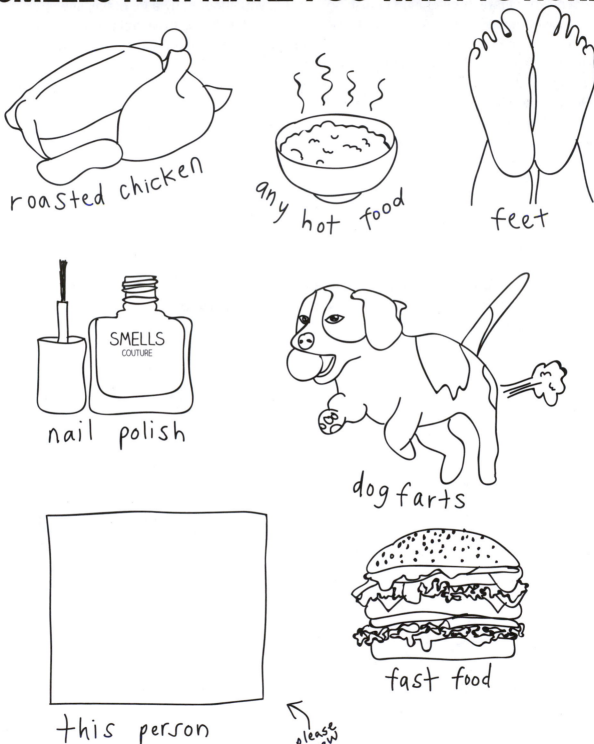

roasted chicken

any hot food

feet

nail polish

SMELLS COUTURE

dog farts

this person

please draw

fast food

# WHERE YOU WERE THE MOMENT YOUR LIFE CHANGED FOREVER

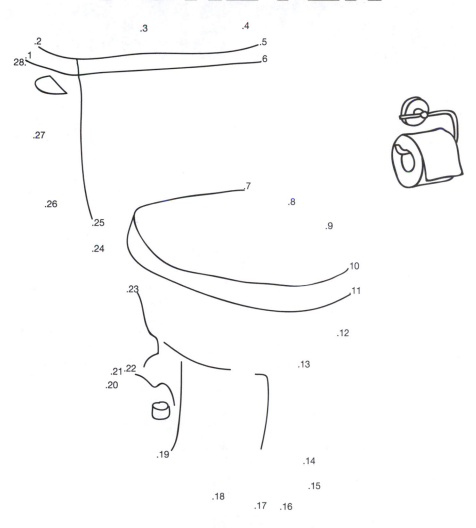

# MATCH THE SONG YOU SHOULD NOT LISTEN TO AND ITS SINGER

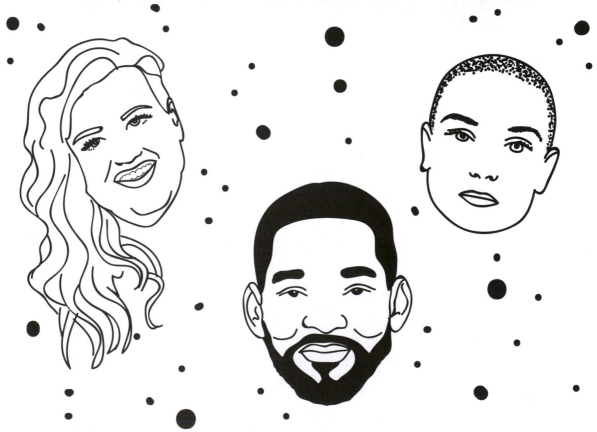

*Ban these songs from your iPod. If one comes on while you're in a Starbucks (while getting a mint tea that you very much wish was an Americano), run. Remember: Tears are only seconds away.*

| | |
|---|---|
| Otis Redding | Father and Son |
| Elton John | Hallelujah |
| Jeff Buckley | Because of You |
| Will Smith | Isn't She Lovely |
| Eric Clapton | Greatest Love of All |
| Fleetwood Mac | Your Song |
| Pearl Jam | Just the Two of Us |
| Cat Power | Nothing Compares 2 U |
| James Taylor | At Last |
| Etta James | That's How Strong My Love Is |
| Nick Drake | I Will Remember You |
| Sarah McLachlan | How Do I Live |
| Stevie Wonder | Over the Rainbow |
| Luther Vandross | Pink Moon |
| Cat Stevens | Landslide |
| Harry Chapin | To Zion |
| LeAnn Rimes | Dance with My Father |
| Whitney Houston | Fire and Rain |
| Sinéad O'Connor | Sea of Love |
| Kelly Clarkson | Tears in Heaven |
| Lauryn Hill | Cat's in the Cradle |
| Judy Garland | Last Kiss |

# THESE SONGS ARE ALSO BANNED:

_____

_____

_____

_____

# WORD ASSOCIATION TIME!

*Write down the first word that comes to mind when you read each of the below.*

Pregnancy: _____

Body: _____

Free time: _____

Sleep: _____

Sex: _____

Bed: _____

Clothing: _____

Layette: _____

Red meat: _____

Chicken: _____

Vegetables: _____

French fries: _____

Labor: _____

Birth: _____

Doctor: _____

Epidural: _____

Mom: _____

Dad: _____

Baby: _____

Doing this exercise made me feel _____. Clearly, I am in need of a little more _____.

# DEAR DIARY,

Oh man, I am so excited to be pregnant. I've been doing so much to prepare! Every day, I do at least 100 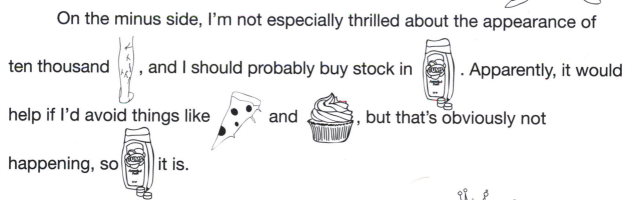, and I've been trying to get to 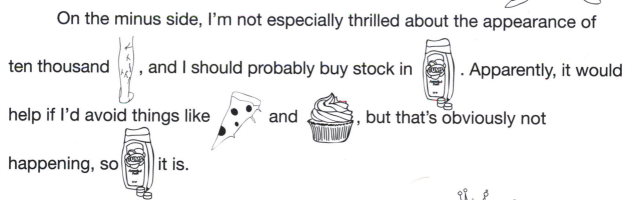 as often as possible. I've also been working on my 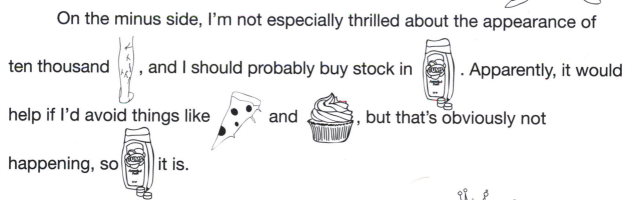 and trying to figure out whether I should actually eat my 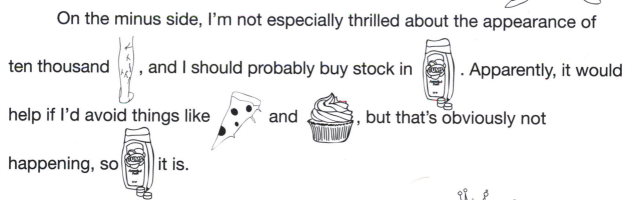. Hmm.

Of course, like any mom-to-be, I spend way too much time poking around on 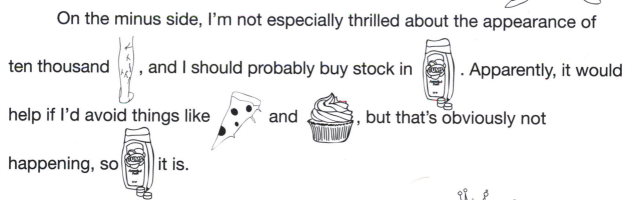. Apparently, the best way to give birth is to 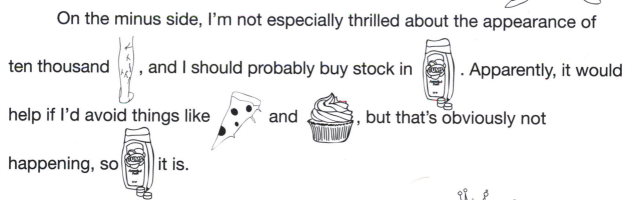. Whatever works, I guess!

On the minus side, I'm not especially thrilled about the appearance of ten thousand 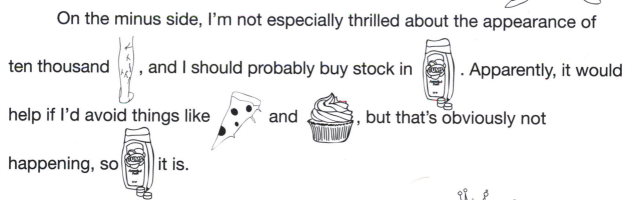, and I should probably buy stock in 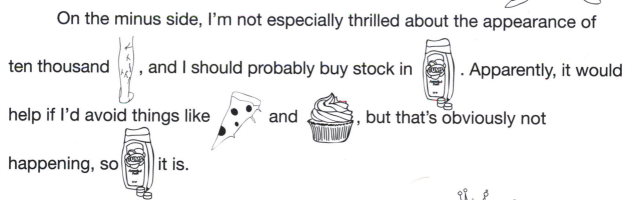. Apparently, it would help if I'd avoid things like 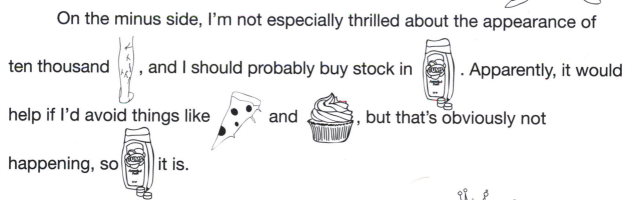 and 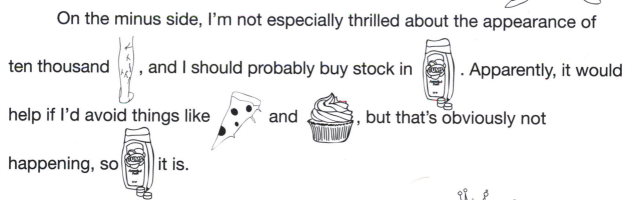, but that's obviously not happening, so 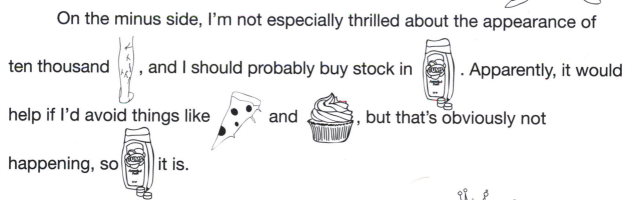 it is.

My 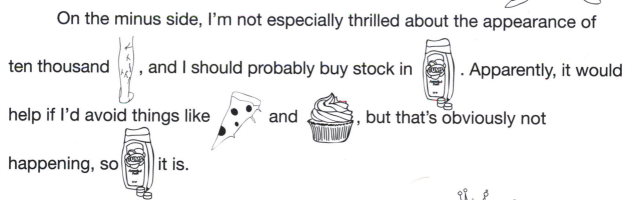 can't come soon enough! (Except for the 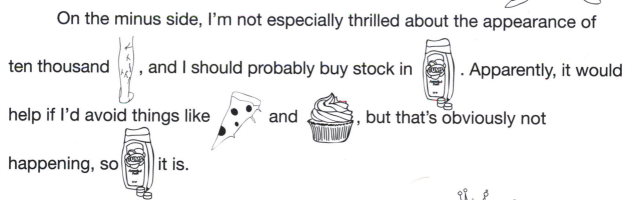 part. That I'm cool with waiting for.)

—Me

**PICTURES:** Kegels, yoga, birth plan, placenta, the Internet, squat, varicose veins, Tums, pizza, cupcakes, Tums, due date, crowning

23

# FIRST TRIMESTER CHECK-IN

I am _____ weeks pregnant.

According to the Internet, my baby is the size of a(n) _____.

This makes me feel _____.

I only want to wear _____.

The part/s of my body that is/are annoying me the most is/are my _____.

I really love my _____, though.

If I even think about _____, I want to throw up.

The biggest to-do on my checklist is _____.

The best thing that happened this week was _____.

The worst thing that happened this week was _____.

When I think about my partner, the primary word that comes to mind is _____.

I really miss _____.

I'm so excited to _____.

When I put my hands on my stomach, I think _____.

Mostly I feel pretty _____.

I want to eat _____ RIGHT NOW.

# YOUR BABY'S DEVELOPMENT

**Week 4**: Your baby has just moved into his new house (at least for the next nine months), aka the amniotic sac. Cozy!

**Week 8**: Your baby looks like an itty-bitty dinosaur with webbed hands and the tiniest fingernails you can possibly imagine. He is also busy kicking and swimming inside you, like a miniature T. rex triathlete minus the bicycle.

**Week 12**: Your baby is starting to look slightly less alien-ish, thanks to ears and eyes that are moving closer to their final positions.

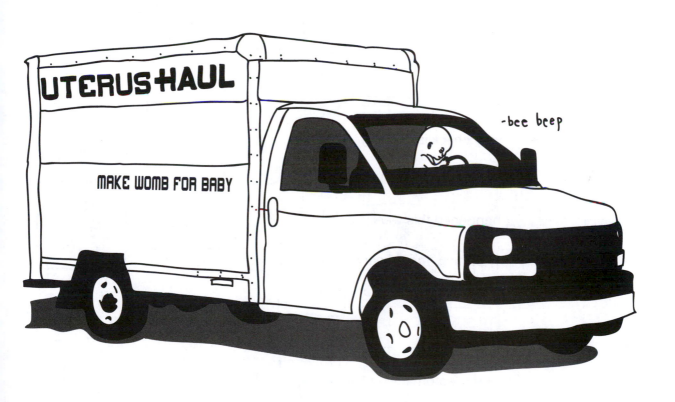

# MAKE IT FROM YOUR DESK TO THE BATHROOM WITHOUT THROWING UP

AVOID CHATTY COWORKERS! A RINGING PHONE! A STINKY TUNA SANDWICH! A TRAY OF DONUTS! A MILLION EMAILS!

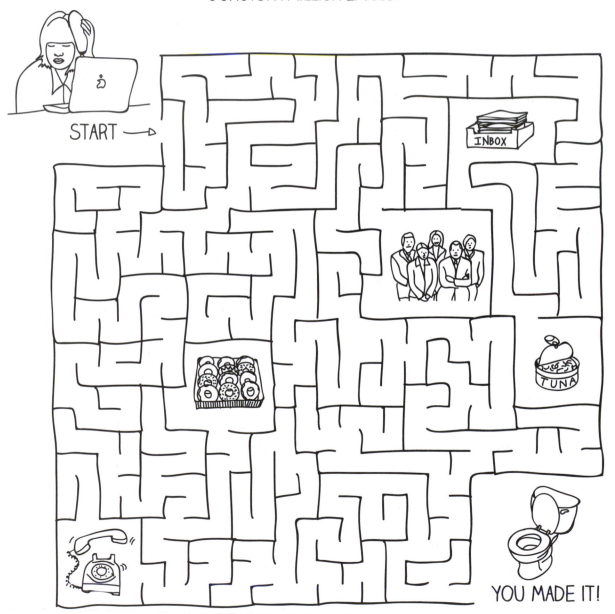

START →

INBOX

TUNA

YOU MADE IT!

# HOW MANY WORDS CAN YOU MAKE OUT OF THE LETTERS IN

## "OH SHIT, I'M PREGNANT"

Nightmare
Migraine

Is that the baby? Is that the heartbeat? Is that a penis? Why do I suddenly have a moustache, and can you please fix this? Why can I not sleep anymore, and can you please fix this? Why am I all of a sudden occasionally vomiting into my own mouth, and can you please fix this? How bad is it if I forget to take my prenatal vitamin sort of all the time? If we have sex, can we, you know ... poke ... the baby? Like is there even the vaguest, most one-in-a-million chance of this happening? So it's still okay to have sex? Do I have to tell my partner that it's still okay to have sex? Can we say I'm not allowed to have sex again until the baby is two years old? Do you have a cell phone number for emergencies? How late is too late to call you? But if it's really an emergency, I can call you whenever? This is a normal amount of weight gain, right? My breasts are going to go back to normal, right? My vagina is going to go back to normal, right? On a scale of one to ten, how bad is coffee actually?

# THINGS EVERY OB ON THE PLANET HAS BEEN ASKED BY NEWLY PREGNANT WOMEN

Ma'am, I'm just the receptionist.

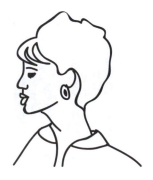

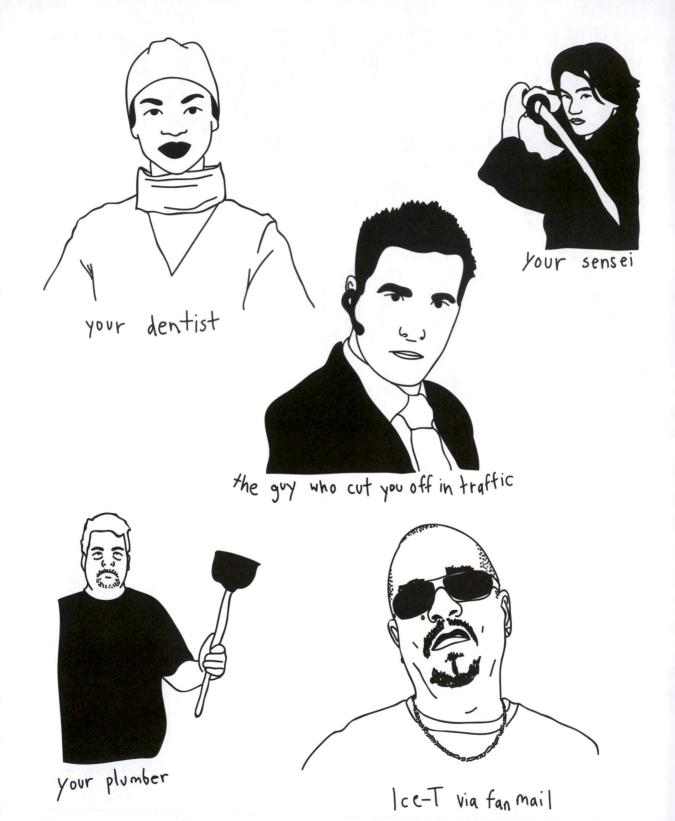

your dentist

your sensei

the guy who cut you off in traffic

your plumber

Ice-T via fan mail

30

# TOP FIVE

## WHO DID YOU TELL ABOUT YOUR PREGNANCY FIRST?

1. _____

2. _____

3. _____

4. _____

5. _____

*Journal:*

**Everyone else in my life found out because:**
   a) I told them
   b) They guessed
   c) I drank a ginger ale in front of them

**I wish I had announced my pregnancy by:**
   a) Doing that thing where you put a baked bun in your home oven and have your partner open it and revel in your adorableness
   b) Doing that thing where you wrap a jar of Prego and give it to your partner and revel in your adorableness
   c) Doing anything other than what I actually did, which was run out of the bathroom with a pee stick in my hand screaming, "HOLY SHIT, WE'RE HAVING A BABY!!!"

# WHO, ME? PREGNANT?!

Not in the mood to let people know you're pregnant yet? While some people wouldn't notice even if you were physically in the middle of the birthing process, others will know the second they see you turn down a cup of coffee or a glass of cabernet. Here's how to keep even your nosiest friends and family members guessing until you're ready to share.

## HOW TO HIDE YOUR PREGNANCY AT A BAR:

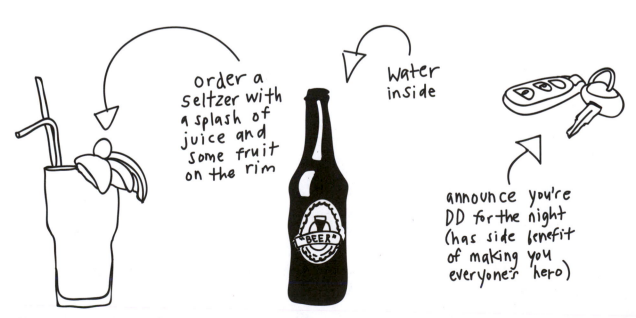

order a seltzer with a splash of juice and some fruit on the rim

water inside

announce you're DD for the night (has side benefit of making you everyone's hero)

# AT A COFFEE SHOP:

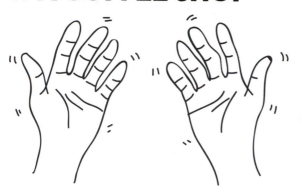

Oh my god, I'm already so over-caffeinated, I couldn't possibly have another!

# AT A SUSHI RESTAURANT:

try a non-raw or vegetarian bento box

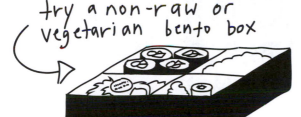

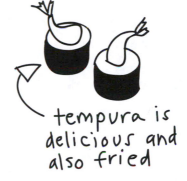

tempura is delicious and also fried

# WHILE SWIMSUIT SHOPPING:

yell distracting things

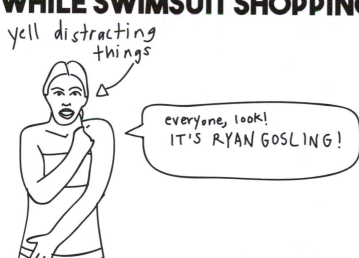

everyone, look! IT'S RYAN GOSLING!

P.S. None of the above applies to any female who is currently pregnant. She has baby radar, and she will know.

# A KITTEN FOR YOU TO COLOR WHILE YOU SIT AROUND CONSTIPATED

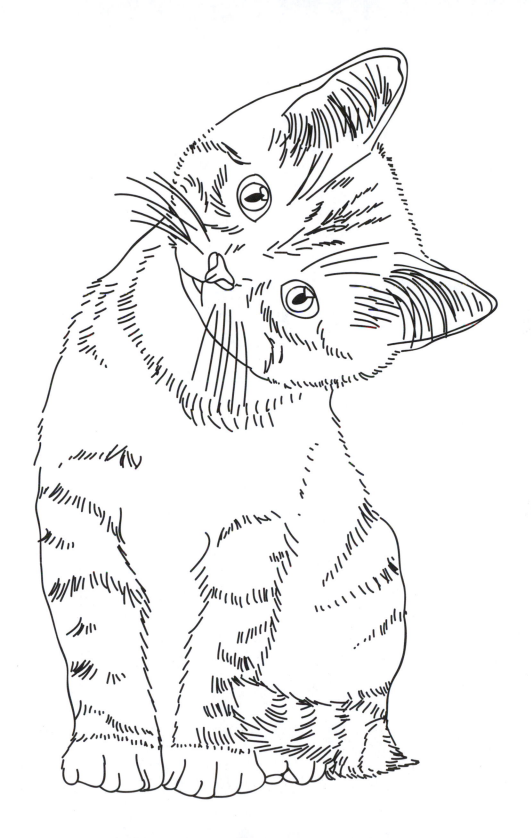

35

# I AM A FERTILITY GODDESS

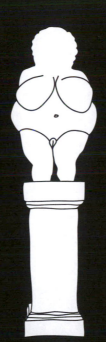

## THE SECOND TRIMESTER

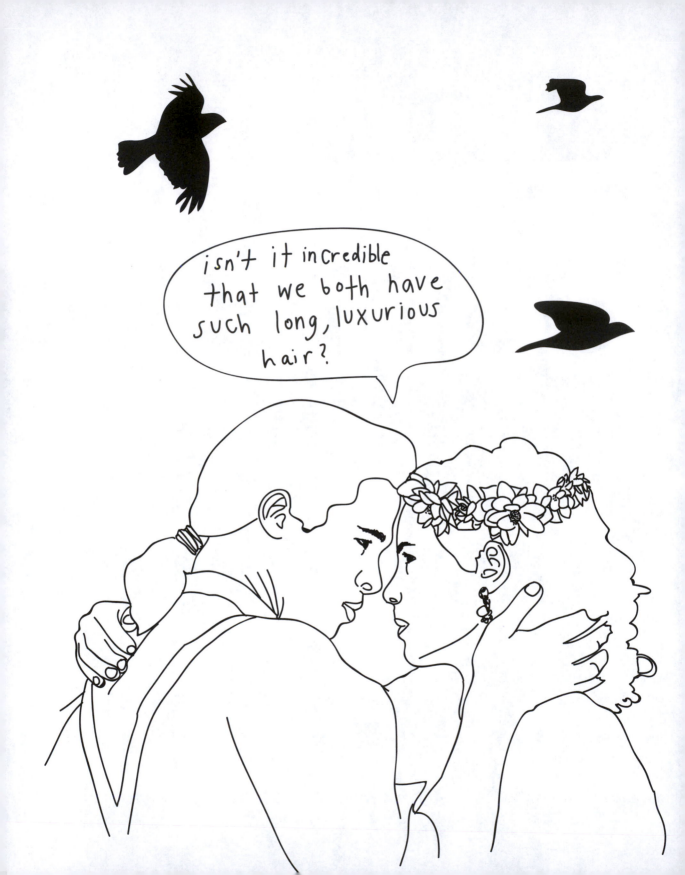

# WELCOME TO THE LAND OF BEING AMAZING

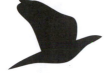

On a scale of 1 to 10, how sick are you of listening to everyone who has ever been pregnant (or known a pregnant person or watched a TV show with a pregnant person in it) tell you how wonderful the second trimester is? How reassured did all these "reassuring statements" make you feel when you were busy wanting to sleep or throw up, or maybe both at the same time?

Well, guess what? All those people were right. (Isn't that annoying?) The second trimester is great and totally makes up for the misery of the first one.

Presenting, a dramatic rendition of your second trimester:

*You step out of a dense fog that smells like feet and emerge onto a sun-drenched plain where Legends of the Fall–era Brad Pitt is standing with his arms outstretched. You float toward him, a flock of adorable little cartoon budgies chirping at your side. Your hair is long and flowing, bedecked with a crown of lotus flowers. You take a deep, meditative breath (because your stomach has not yet moved your lungs into your shoulders, and you can still do this), and you do not sneeze. In the second trimester, there is no pollen.*

If we have not yet made this clear, the second trimester includes some extremely good stuff. First, you are basically a hair-and-nail supermodel. The best part, though, is the energy: You will suddenly find yourself behaving like a person who has ingested nine espressos, minus the anxiety and toxic breath.

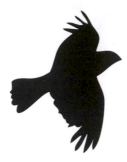

More fun things coming your way:

1. You can finally tell everyone. (Okay, so you already told the mailman, the guy who makes your egg sandwich at the bodega, the Verizon customer service rep, your neighbor's plumber, and the mystery person who picked up the phone when you were trying to call your dentist, but now you can tell your boss and Facebook.)

2. People will start to notice. This is fun, because now they'll start doing things like giving you seats on crowded trains and holding doors for you and generally treating you like a snowflake.

3. You can start planning your shower and choosing stuff for your registry. BUY ALL THE TINY THINGS.

4. You may feel your baby move for the first time. This is 100 percent as thrilling as it sounds. And in just a few short weeks you will enter a period of life during which you enjoy a nightly viewing of The Most Exciting Event That Has Ever Happened: You will start actually seeing the skin on your stomach moving around. You will not be able to believe that this has ever happened to a person before, and you will make a videotape of your stomach and put it on YouTube, where it will get six views because this totally happens to everyone.

5. Sex still feels like a reasonable pastime! You may even find yourself wanting to do it way more than usual (the reason it's so great right now has something to do with increased blood flow to the pertinent areas, but whatever: orgasms).

It's an exciting time—one of the most exciting times of your life. Enjoy. And for god's sake, take a lot of photos.

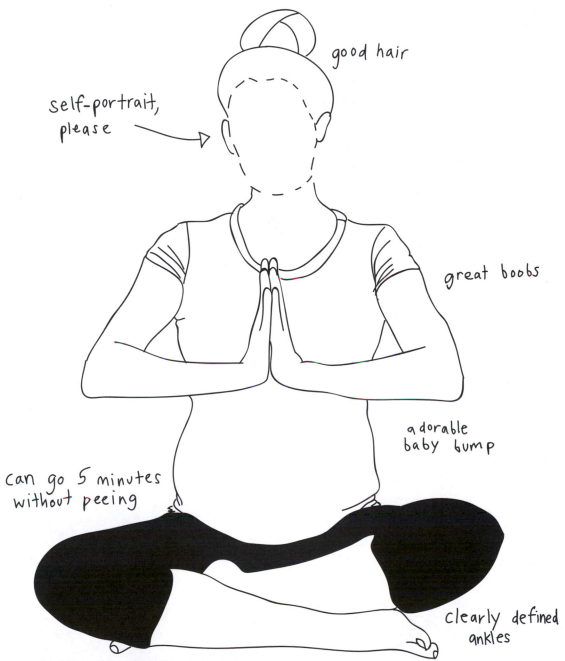

# A PORTRAIT OF YOU IN ALL YOUR GLORY

# DO TELL:

**The best part of the second trimester is:**

a) Telling people I'm pregnant
b) Being treated like I'm pregnant
c) Feeling the baby start to move
d) The hair
e) The nails
f) The sex
g) The energy
h) The purchasing of tiny things
i) All the above
j) Me, generally, because I AM AMAZING

**List five things about you that are absolutely spectacular (we know, it's hard to keep it down to five):**

1. _____

2. _____

3. _____

4. _____

5. _____

# DO NOT READ THESE BOOKS
## (EVEN IF YOUR MOM GIVES THEM TO YOU BECAUSE SHE LOVES YOU)

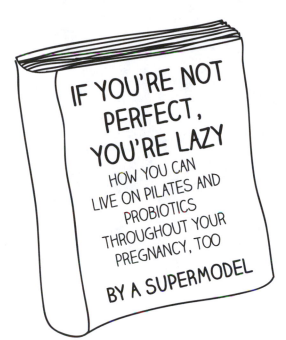

**IF YOU'RE NOT PERFECT, YOU'RE LAZY**

HOW YOU CAN LIVE ON PILATES AND PROBIOTICS THROUGHOUT YOUR PREGNANCY, TOO

**BY A SUPERMODEL**

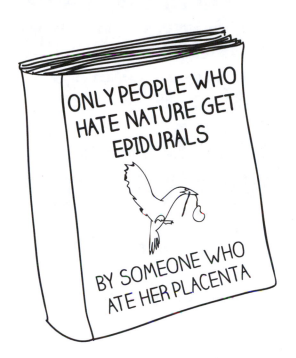

**ONLY PEOPLE WHO HATE NATURE GET EPIDURALS**

BY SOMEONE WHO ATE HER PLACENTA

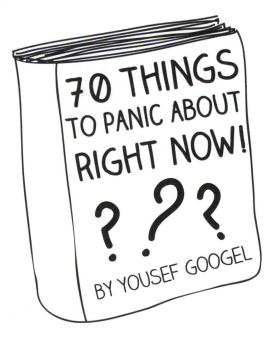

**70 THINGS TO PANIC ABOUT RIGHT NOW!**

**? ? ?**

BY YOUSEF GOOGEL

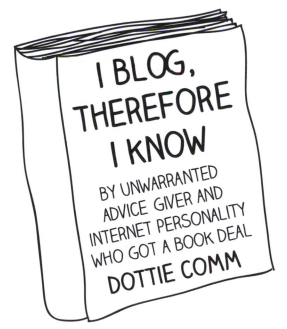

**I BLOG, THEREFORE I KNOW**

BY UNWARRANTED ADVICE GIVER AND INTERNET PERSONALITY WHO GOT A BOOK DEAL

**DOTTIE COMM**

# YOGA TEACHERS (ALSO YOUR MOM FRIENDS, YOUR PARENTS, PEOPLE ON FACEBOOK, ALL ARTICLES, AND EVERYONE YOU MEET) WANT TO TELL YOU HOW TO GIVE BIRTH, BUT YOU DON'T HAVE TO LISTEN

There's something about pregnancy that invites everyone within shooting distance to approach you and ask you very intimate questions. Your mailman wants to know if you plan on a vaginal birth. The lady on line behind you at the movie theater warns you that eating popcorn may affect your child's ability to read the complete works of James Joyce by age three (she read a study, you see). Your yoga teacher stops you mid–downward dog to tell you that (a) she is a doula, (b) you need a doula, (c) you need to do more yoga, and (d) you also need to have a home birth with no drugs and breastfeed until the day your child enrolls in college and also please cut out dairy, okay?

In short: You will be approached almost constantly by near-strangers inquiring about the state of your uterus. Almost all these people mean well, but that doesn't give them the right to invade your privacy.

Maybe you've always envisioned a home birth, just you and your partner and a midwife. Maybe you won't feel safe unless you're in a hospital, knowing that very strong drugs are within arm's reach. Maybe you're too terrified of the whole "birth" thing to even think about it yet. All these options are fine—wonderful, in fact—because however you want or need to give birth is the right way to do it.

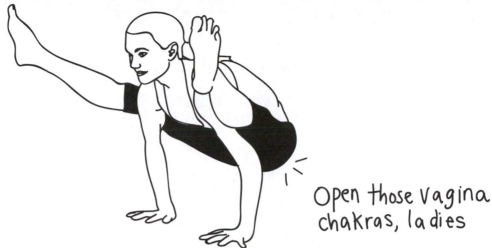

Open those vagina chakras, ladies

Here are some suggested comebacks for your friendly mailman/theatergoer/yoga teacher/ whomever who wants to offer some awesomely helpful advice so that you, too, can give birth exactly the way that they or their partner did (isn't that great?!):

"Jeez, a home birth sounds amazing, but I'm not sure my doctor will approve of me flying back to my planet so late in the third trimester."

"<Shrugs.> You know, I thought about it and I'm just going to do whatever that Duggar lady did."

"I haven't decided what I'm going to do yet, but I should probably take into consideration the fact that I live in a submarine."

"I'm just going to hire a stunt double to take care of the whole thing for me."

**List the strangest or most aggravating suggestions you've received so far:**

_____

_____

_____

_____

_____

# GET FROM ONE SIDE OF THE PARTY TO THE OTHER

AVOID CRUSTY ROOM-TEMPERATURE DIPS! HARD LIQUOR! PEOPLE YOU BARELY KNOW WHO'D LIKE TO TOUCH YOUR STOMACH AND ASK ABOUT THE STATE OF YOUR VAGINA!

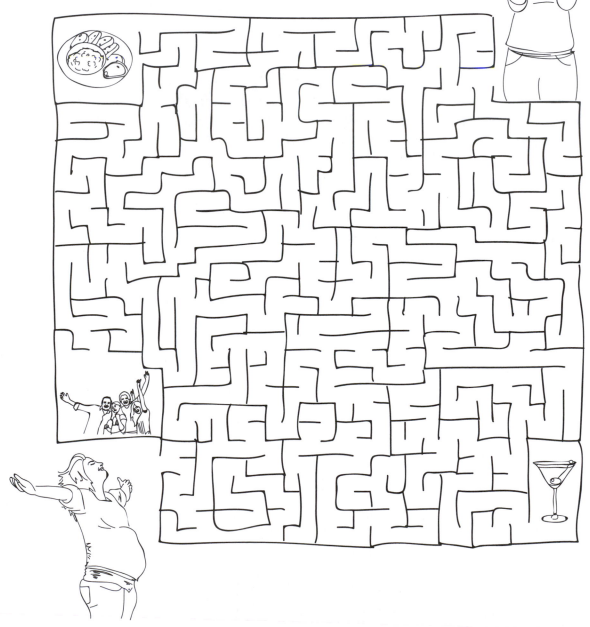

# TILT THE PAGE TO REVEAL A SECRET MESSAGE

# BAD BABY NAMES

*Apparently, the late 1800s/early 1900s were a time of unprecedented inventiveness in the way of bad baby names. These may not have been "popular," but they definitely existed (in 1910, there were nine hundred and ten newborn girls who got stuck with "Classie") and were definitely bestowed upon tiny, innocent babies who—just a guess—later grew up to be very pissed off at their parents. Chestina and Ples: This one's for you.*

AUTHOR
BOBBYE
CARRY
CHESTINA
CHRIST
CLASSIE
COUNCIL
DIMPLE
DOCK
EARLY
FATE
FOUNT

GORGE
GREEN
HILDRED
ICY
LAWYER
LEMON
LITTLE
LOCKIE
MANLEY
MAYO
MURL
ORANGE

OVA
PINKEY
PLEASANT
PLES
ROLLA
SISTER
SON
SPURGEON
SQUIRE
TOY
VESTER
WASH

## Journal:

**Okay, if I had to choose one of these for my own baby, it'd be:**
   a) Mayo, obviously, because mayo is delicious
   b) Rolla, because it sounds pretty badass
   c) Lemon, because it's terrible but also kind of cute
   d) Christ, because why not start the kid off on a high note
   e) Fill in your own: _____

```
E T T K X D N L O K M Y U L B K S A U A T O O S Z O I N Q A
S Y N E E R G I A Y R T P I D E X C K W R M P I R Y F U T Y
S C B A Q A L B M W A U L T Y O T M E X K U F A R Q U O J O
I F V B S E R A Z Y Y M E T C V X Q G I R W N O K P D B P Y
C N E F O A I A Y E B E S L Q I M D R G R G E U C N W N H U
H B L E Q B E L O K Q X R E M B B Y E C E T Y O O K F A T E
Y K P M O L A L T N J K I I B G G O P N F O J N D U H V H C
V E F K F J F O P I V B R X F M N W B O I Y H Y D V W R V L
N P L Q J Q R R P P I P T W I K T N R U X Q R S X K O Y G E
I X W N X M L M O D V P U E Y A N I T S E H C Q U T U U N I
G B U I A L Y G P B P U Y Y J T K W J R A B B U G O A U H Y
C R B Z O M E O T S V C E U B L O I S Y W F F I N G E F R A
P Y T C C A L E W N I F Z J O Q K B T M O V D R N M M R E P
T J K P R H N A P Y M Z G R K J C K R M H L X E U N A P J V
G I B L Z G O N V J K M B M T R A Y H Z J V T F T C K W Z N
E T Y G M E S G V G K R E T S I S R E T S E V S L A G W Z A
J P Y U F Y P P P V B P L B E W W D F G R L I O V E K B M B
U U R D Y C K R C F C L A S S I E G W W O R V O S L M Z V U
D L R C E B L P U A E T N P E P Q J Y L H B T D A W U R P A
C I X T E V I V B E L G V A R L U U V C V H L P R Z C P R D
H Q M T C Q W G O M K D H Z V J L J K P E C E S Q L M K A E
W M O P F L K C O X A M O U V Z P M T Q K P M W C Y S N A R
M G S L L S M H N R T V L C B L C Q O R L R O P M M Q V V D
F O U N T E S R K P G I J V Y F Z T C F X H N T X B J H G L
A J P E X A T Z X M C E Y S B I X N R E G D D G B W S Q X I
Q V X W W A E V R N A U T H O R Y M V E G N I D K D A M J H
K F O I T U O V U V F W Q K R G M D R N Y E Q W O Q M R E Y
T U K U R T Q O Y S N B U E J W L H B Z A H C T C Z O F O H
U G N K S F C S T C V V T G E M E A Z B K Q L C L C L K S S L E
H L J K B F Z Z D P B Z N L V C G L Q N R I Y F C Y N D O C
```

49

# TIME TO BUST OUT

## WHERE WILL YOU GO ON YOUR BABYMOON?

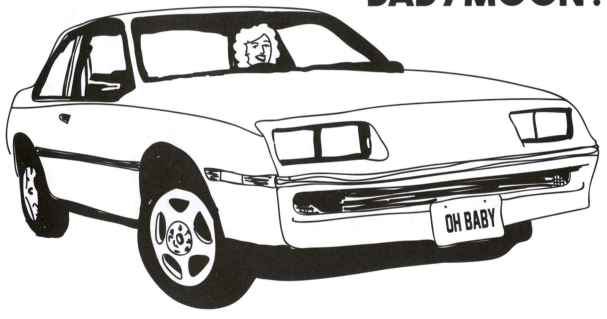

_____

_____

_____

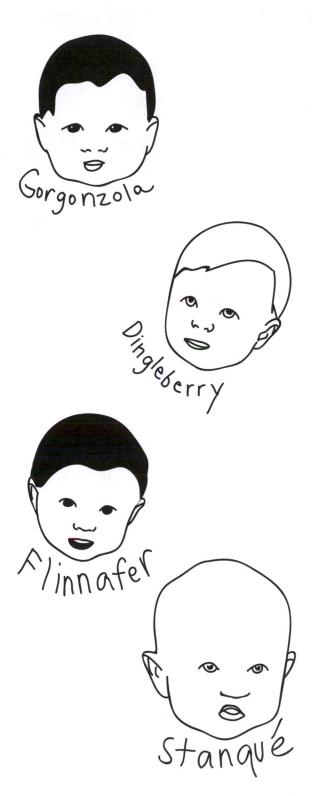

Gorgonzola

Dingleberry

Flinnafer

Stanqué

# LET'S NAME THIS KID!

Here is the problem with choosing a baby name: Whatever you choose, someone very close to you (and definitely your mother and/or mother-in-law) is going to hate it, and they are going to tell you so. So what you have to do is either (a) not tell anyone until the name is inscribed on the birth certificate and part of public record forever and ever, or (b) not care what anyone else thinks. We recommend the latter.

In the meantime, though, you're probably going to have to come to something approaching "agreement" with your partner, because while you're the one who will be physically removing a child from your body and thus totally get the last word on everything, for the rest of your life, it's nice to let them think they have a say.

So grab a couple of pens and sit down together, and let's get this kid named.

1. Which of these categories appeals to you? Circle all that apply, and have your partner circle all the ones that he or she likes in a different color.

WHIMSICAL         CLASSIC

EXTREMELY UNUSUAL    HIPSTER

GREEK MYTH         INTERNATIONAL

OLD-FASHIONED      NATURE

2. Keeping the categories that you *both* like in mind, list ten names each. Free associate! Get weird! Anything goes.

**Me**

1._____
2._____
3._____
4._____
5._____
6._____
7._____
8._____
9._____
10._____

**My Partner**

1._____
2._____
3._____
4._____
5._____
6._____
7._____
8._____
9._____
10._____

3. Now cross out any names on your partner's list that you can't even begin to handle because they are so terrible, and have him or her do the same. (If you get annoyed, just remember: You own The Vagina, and if you want to name your child "Spicy," that is what is going to happen.)

4. Cross out any names that remind either of you of ex-boyfriends or ex-girlfriends.

5. Cross out the names of anyone who was mean to either of you in elementary school.

6. Now circle any of the names on your partner's list that you can live with, and have him or her do the same. Write each of the mutually agreed upon names below next to the last name you're planning to use, and hop online to find each first name's meaning.

| First Name | Last Name | First Name's Meaning |
|---|---|---|
|  |  |  |
|  |  |  |
|  |  |  |
|  |  |  |
|  |  |  |

7. Cross out all the names that sound creepy with your last name (no Ben Dovers or Seymour Weiners, please).

8. Cross out all the names that have meanings that either of you cannot live with.

And ta daaa! Now you should either have a couple of names that you both like, or none at all. (Either way, that was kind of fun, right?)

P.S. Please name your baby "Spicy."

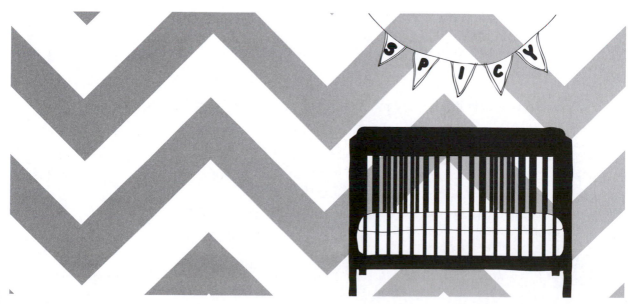

# Quiz

# MIND THOSE MANNERS

You may think you've got a handle on this whole "how to act like a human being in society" thing, but with the arrival of a very small yet very loud person who is completely uninterested in excreting substances in appropriate places, all bets are off.

*Find out just how well prepared you are to handle the (many, many) messy situations that are about to come your way.*

1. Over the first year of my child's life, it is a virtual certainty that he or she will vomit:
   a) In the car seat
   b) At a restaurant while seated next to a couple who is clearly on a first date
   c) On you and/or your hair (many, many times)
   d) All the above

2. When a stranger asks you when you're due and you've already had the baby, the correct response is to:
   a) Giggle and change the subject
   b) Politely correct them
   c) Not-so-politely correct them
   d) Side-eye, all the way

3. Which of the below is it *not* okay to say to your partner while in the throes of labor?
   a) Go. Away.
   b) GET ME DRUGS
   c) We are never having sex again
   d) You're not even the father!

4. If your child spits up on your new-mom friend's shirt, you should:
   a) Apologize your little heart out
   b) Offer to buy her a new top
   c) Worry that she will no longer want to be friends with you
   d) Pass a wipe her way

5. If you are on a plane and your child has a meltdown, the best response is to:
   a) Give him a bottle; it might just be that his ears aren't clearing
   b) At least look like you're putting a massive amount of effort into resolving the situation
   c) Have a good cry yourself
   d) Cocktails for everyone!

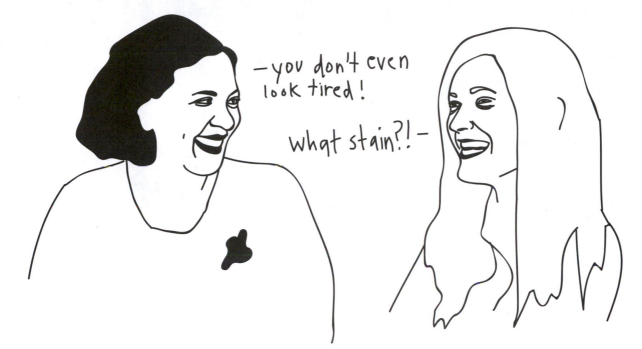

—you don't even look tired!

what stain?!—

# answers

1. (d) Your child will throw up everywhere. Constantly. And mostly in places where you really, seriously do not want him to. Carry wipes.

2. Well, technically you should do (b), because you're a grown-up, but let's get real: (c) and (d) are both totally acceptable alternatives, because if you reference a total stranger's pregnancy and she is not at that moment running down the street waving a sign that says "THERE IS A BABY IN MY UTERUS," you deserve to be made to feel uncomfortable. Side-eye away.

3. (d) You probably shouldn't say this, because even if it happens to be true, it might make said person less likely to bring you ice chips and make sure your birthing playlist is in working order. And while (c) may actually be true, best not to ruin the surprise before you have to.

4. (d) But the truth is you probably don't need to do anything if this happens to another new mom because she didn't notice. And if she did notice, she didn't care.

5. All these are excellent ideas.

# SOME TIPS FOR YOUR PREGNANCY PHOTOS

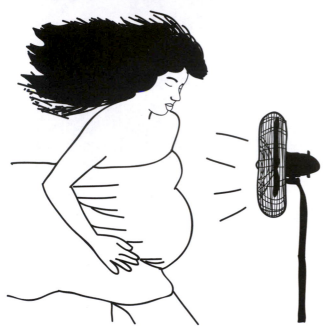

take it easy with the wind machine

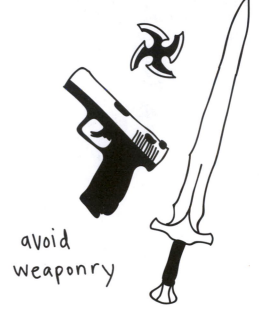

avoid weaponry

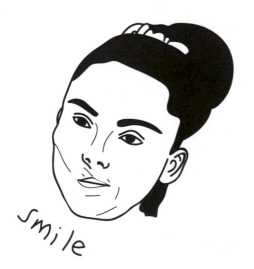

smile

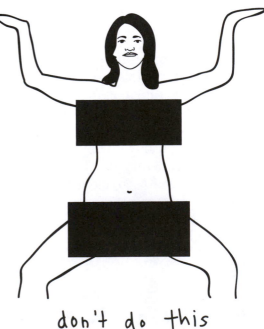

don't do this

# UNCONVENTIONAL MOBILE IDEAS

Let's get one thing straight right off the bat: Your newborn does not care about his mobile, because he cannot see more than six inches in front of his face. Even when he does start seeing, he still doesn't care about the Mozart-playing baby elephants that you so lovingly hung in his direct line of sight; the speck on the wall over there is just as interesting.

That said, if you feel the urgent need to express yourself in mobile form, why not go the DIY route? Dangling rain-forest creatures or your college wine cork collection; it's pretty much all the same to him.

Here are some mobile ideas for the more "experimental" among you.

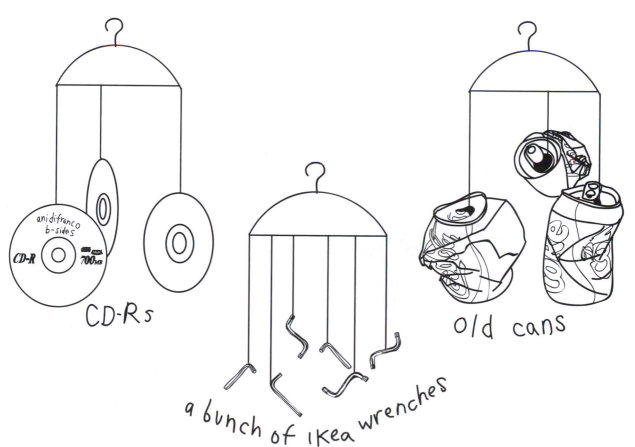

CD-Rs

a bunch of ikea wrenches

old cans

# THE PINTEREST

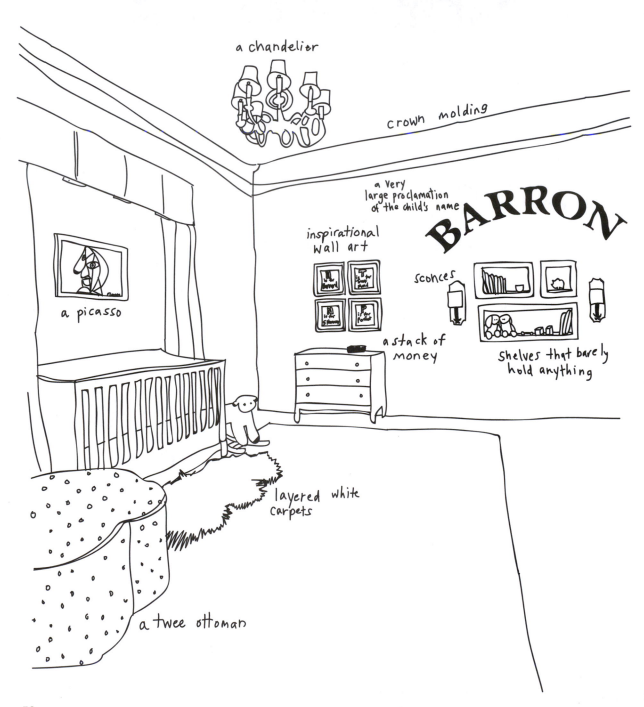

a chandelier

crown molding

a very
large proclamation
of the child's name

BARRON

inspirational
wall art

a picasso

sconces

a stack of
money

shelves that barely
hold anything

layered white
carpets

a twee ottoman

# NURSERY

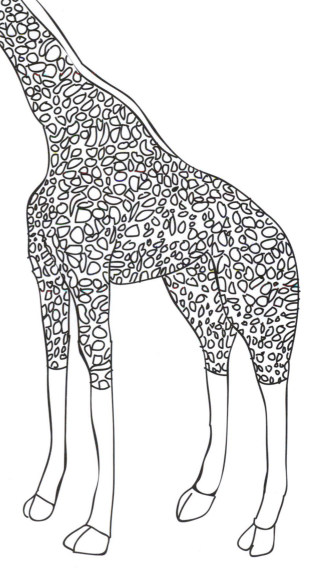

While Pinterest's stated purpose is, of course, "inspiration," the site's true function is to make all who gaze upon its endless feed of perfect pie crusts and Beyoncé's hair realize that we are wildly inadequate in virtually every area of our existence. On Pinterest, you can discover just how many things about you are lacking, from your nail polish application skills to your window treatments to your ability to artfully light and photograph your dinner.

For moms-to-be, however, the primary goal of Pinterest is to drive home the realization that your life — and certainly your baby's life — will not be complete without an organic Moses basket and an artfully arranged wall of reclaimed wood squares hand-painted with encouraging messages, feathers, and arrows. (And a chandelier over the crib, but that goes without saying.)

All that's well and good, but why not branch out?

# DÉCOR INSPIRATION FOR THE PINTEREST-AVERSE

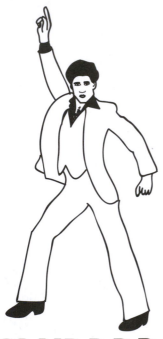

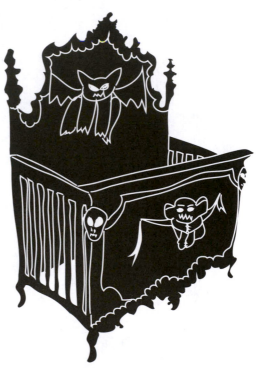

## CLURRRB

Look, you two are going to be partying all night anyway, so why not make the nursery somewhere you want to hang out and have a little fun? You're going to need a serious sound system and a TV with the full run of *The Bad Girls Club* loaded into it. Disco ball and life-size John Travolta cutout optional but obviously recommended.

## GOTH

You know what a pitch-black room is? A room in which there is nothing to do except SLEEP. And when babies sleep, all is well with the world. So how about a room with black walls, black furniture, a black rug, and blackout curtains? You say "morbid," we say "zzzzzzz."

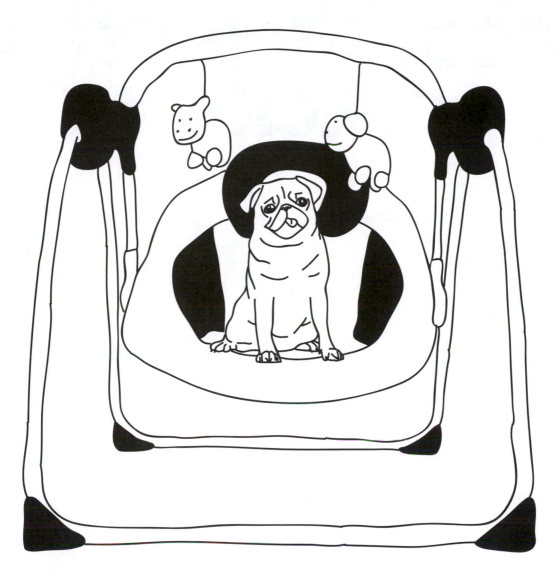

# DOG–HAIR CHIC

Also known as "I fucking give up," this chic and calming space
features four to seven piles of unfolded laundry for collapsing
into, an elegantly stacked trio of Costco-size diaper boxes, a rug
overlaid with a whisper-soft layer of pet hair, and a copy of *What
to Expect When You're Expecting* that has been cried on.

# SECOND TRIMESTER
# CHECK-IN

I am _____ weeks pregnant.

According to the Internet, my baby is the size of a/n _____.

This makes me feel _____.

I only want to wear _____.

The part/s of my body that is/are annoying me the most is/are my _____.

I really love my _____, though.

If I even think about _____, I want to throw up.

The biggest to-do on my checklist right now is _____.

The best thing that happened this week was _____.

The worst thing that happened this week was _____.

When I think about my partner, the primary word that comes to mind is _____.

I really miss _____.

I'm so excited to _____.

The baby's movements remind me of _____.

Mostly I feel pretty _____.

I want to eat _____ RIGHT NOW.

# YOUR BABY'S DEVELOPMENT

**Week 14:** Your baby can make expressions and is primarily using them to frown and grimace, thereby getting some early practice for his teenage years.

**Week 19:** Your baby has hair! Sort of. More like a very, very tiny buzz cut.

**Week 22:** Your baby still has wrinkly, raisin-y old-man skin, but she'll start gaining weight and filling out soon.

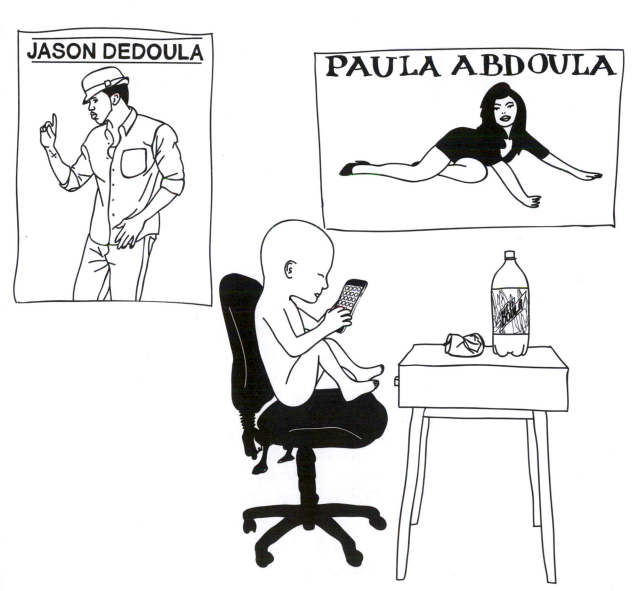

# HOW TO REGISTER WITHOUT CRYING

When you take your first step into a Baby Stuff Store, all moderately pregnant and wide-eyed and defenseless, you know what the salesperson sees? Lunch.

Beware the salesperson in the Baby Stuff Store. Oh sure, he is very kind and helpful, but there is a big sign on your forehead that says I HAVE NO IDEA WHAT I'M DOING, and he just spotted it. And the next thing that he is going to do is hand you a list of items that you absolutely must purchase if you love your child. (…You do love your child, don't you?)

You will recognize the names of about one percent of the items on this list, and the total price will be at least one million dollars. He will then explain to you how vital it is that you purchase not only the ExerSaucer, but also the bouncy seat, the play gym, and the vibrating egg that is more technologically advanced than your car and will lull your child to sleep by precisely re-creating the movements of a tree swing, a car ride, or a kangaroo—it's up to you! Didn't you know that your infant must have multiple brightly colored surfaces upon which to not move in order to acquire those crucial early developmental skills? You didn't?! (Good luck with that Harvard application, then.)

You will look at the price tags of these items. You will mentally calculate the square footage of your living space. And then you will cry.

But it doesn't have to go down that way! Try these things instead:

## 1. **Cheat**

Ask your friends who already have babies (especially the ones who have more than one) to send you their own registry lists. Here's the key: Ask them to cross out anything they ended up not needing and to add the items that ended up being lifesavers.

## 2. **Just Say No to Cashmere**

If you absolutely cannot live without overpriced baby clothing, go to a baby consignment shop. They are full of ridiculously fancy baby items that nobody ever used, because nobody ever uses ridiculously fancy baby items. Because what babies do to these items is destroy them. You won't use them either, but one of the fun parts of pregnancy is that you get to make irrational purchasing choices and no one can get mad at you because you are making a human being from scratch and are thus basically a goddess.

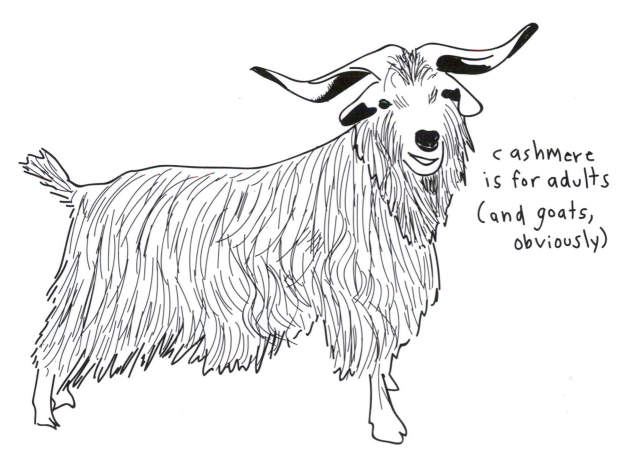

cashmere is for adults (and goats, obviously)

### 3. Mooch Off Your Friends

Your friends who already have children have so much stuff. They do not want it in their houses. If they are not having more children, they will probably just give it to you. If they are thinking of having more children, they will probably give it to you on the condition that you give it back to them when you're done. You have a village: Use it.

### 4. Remember That Adding the Word "Baby" to a Product Also Adds Approximately Five Dollars to Its Price Tag

You know what a "baby washcloth" is? A washcloth. Except it might have a duck on it. Your baby does not care.

### 5. Register Online

If you register online, you can avoid (a) guilt-inducing salespeople and (b) crying over how adorable and tiny everything is (so tiny, so cute, oh my god I'm having a babyyyyy…).

P.S. Keep your receipts, because babies may be tiny and cute, but they are also picky little assholes.

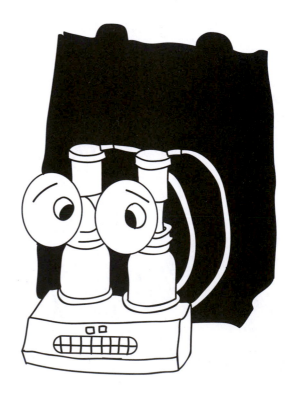

Will you register for this ~~milk monster~~ breast pump?

# GET TO THE CHECKOUT AT BABIES "R" US

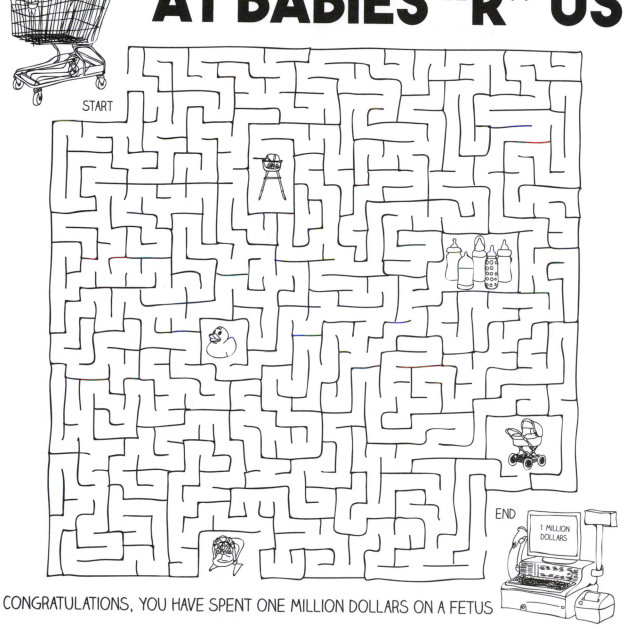

START

END

1 MILLION DOLLARS

CONGRATULATIONS, YOU HAVE SPENT ONE MILLION DOLLARS ON A FETUS

# THINGS PEOPLE TELL YOU YOUR BABY NEEDS THAT YOUR BABY DOES NOT NEED

Every mom you know will have a lot of advice for you about what worked for their babies. This is good information, so lock it away somewhere. Please also know that almost none of these things will work for your baby. Swaddlers, blankets, pacifiers, bottles, even types of clothing: These are all subject to your baby's persnickety little preferences. Don't buy a whole bunch of Velcro swaddlers only to find that your baby can't stand them, or ten newborn onesies with snaps before realizing that you prefer zippers. If you aren't sure: Wait, and then Amazon.

## 1. A Wipe Warmer

This is a thing that you buy for $20 and then put your wipes in and plug into the wall, in order to warm wipes. Another (free) option for wipe warming is "scrunch the wipe in your hand for five seconds." Also, learning an analog technique means that you can change the baby anywhere that is not your home without stunning them with the arctic blast of an unwarmed wipe. (And even if you don't warm up your wipes at all, your baby still won't suffer the very rare disease of icicle ass.)

## 2. A Bottle Warmer

By the time you read all the instructions and figure out what level you need to boop it on and for how many minutes for however many ounces you mixed or pumped, you could have warmed it in the sink with hot water. Spend that $30 on an hour of babysitting and a large pizza instead.

## 3. Baby Shoes

Babies do not walk. People who do not walk do not need shoes.

## 4. Expensive Burp Cloths

Let's be clear: These are for you. If you want your child to vomit on tiny quilted elephants, that's totally fine, but your baby seriously does not care. Get the massive bag of cheap white raglike ones and fling them about with joyful abandon, knowing that each one did not cost you the equivalent of four Starbucks lattes (you will need the lattes more).

## 5. Anything from Restoration Hardware

Everything is triple-washed organic hand-sewn linen-blend alpaca, sure, but you know what it really is? Very, very expensive stuff for your baby to destroy. Don't do it.

# MATCH THE ORGAN TO ITS BRAND-NEW LOCATION

Did you know that your small intestine is 22 feet long? Where does that even go? Find out with this exercise, which will also help you understand why you can't stop peeing.

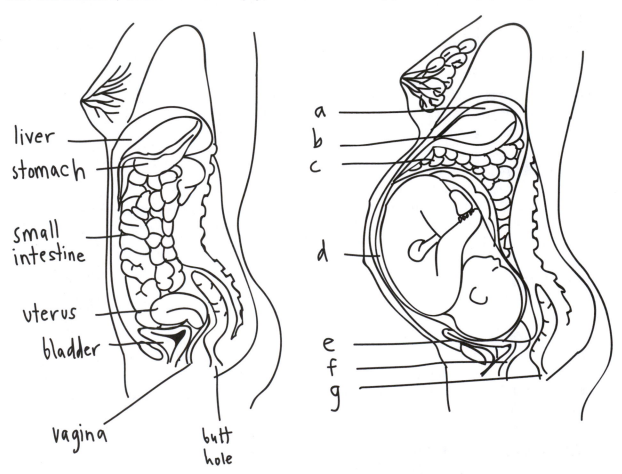

liver
stomach
small intestine
uterus
bladder
vagina
butt hole

a
b
c
d
e
f
g

# TOP FIVE

## WHAT ARE YOUR FAVORITE THINGS TO WEAR RIGHT NOW?

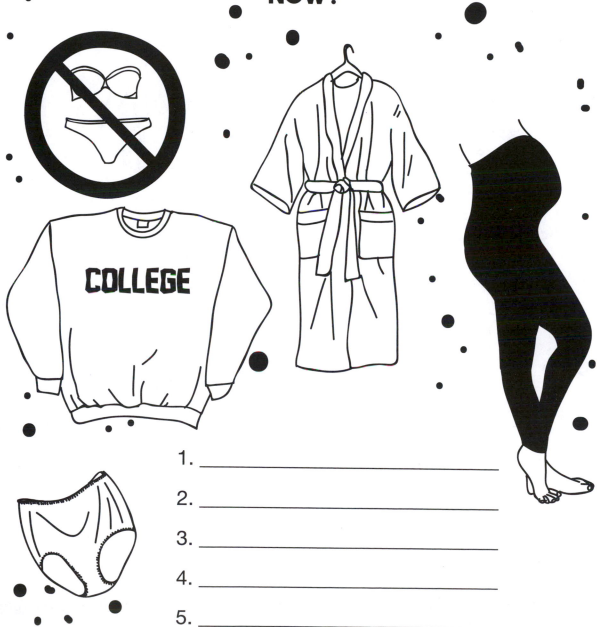

1. _____
2. _____
3. _____
4. _____
5. _____

# WHICH $1500 STROLLER IS DIFFERENT?

Bonus: Which $1500 stroller would your baby not puke on/crush Cheerios into?

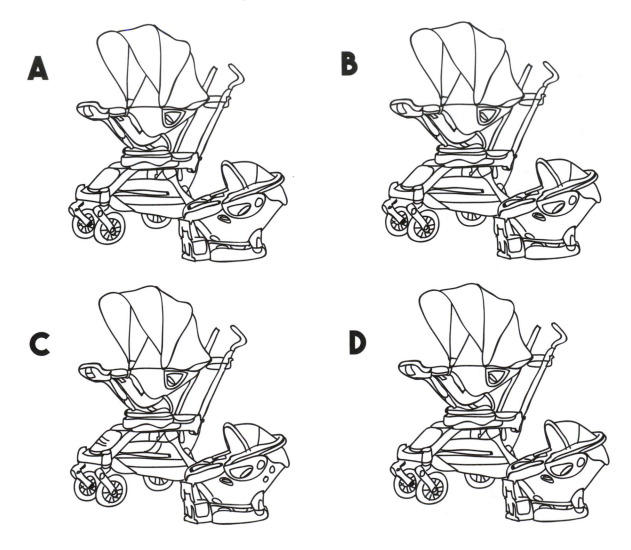

A

B

C

D

# UNSCRAMBLE YOUR PREGNANCY SYMPTOMS

*Unscramble the letters to reveal the "exciting" bodily changes you can expect in the second trimester.*

**1. DUMBNEGLIGES**

\_ \_ \_ \_ \_ \_ \_ \_ \_ \_ \_ \_

**2. BLESSDONEE**

\_ \_ \_ \_ \_ \_ \_ \_

**3. AGRACEDLAVISHING**

\_ \_ \_ \_ \_ \_ \_ \_ \_ \_ \_ \_ \_ \_ \_

**4. CANTEENGINSPOT**

\_ \_ \_ \_ \_ \_ \_ \_ \_ \_ \_ \_ \_ \_

**5. AHWIDERSIR**

\_ \_ \_ \_ \_ \_ \_ \_ \_

**6. NECKGNUIQI**

\_ \_ \_ \_ \_ \_ \_ \_ \_ \_

**7. CAVEREVISIONS**

\_ \_ \_ \_ \_ \_ \_ \_ \_ \_ \_ \_

**8. BARHENRUT**

\_ \_ \_ \_ \_ \_ \_ \_

# 4 SUPERFOODS YOU HAVE TO EAT RIGHT NOW

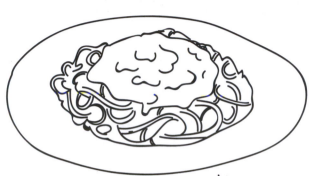

a never-ending pasta bowl (with chia seeds sprinkled on top)

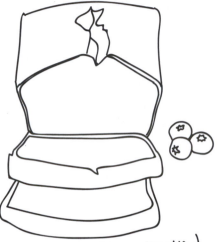

an entire pound cake (and a couple of blueberries)

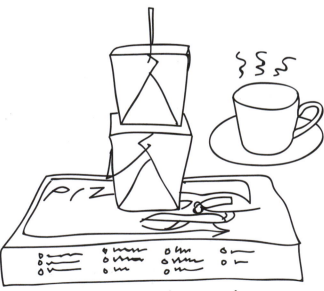

Chinese food on pizza (with raspberry leaf tea on the side)

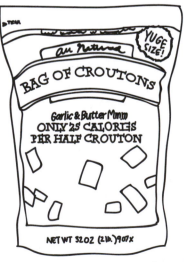

BAG OF CROUTONS

Garlic & Butter Mmm
ONLY 25 CALORIES
PER HALF CROUTON

YUGE SIZE!

au Natural

NET WT 32OZ (2lb.)907x

a ~~kale salad~~ bag of croutons

# GET THE BOX OF PASTRIES HOME WITHOUT EATING THEM ALL

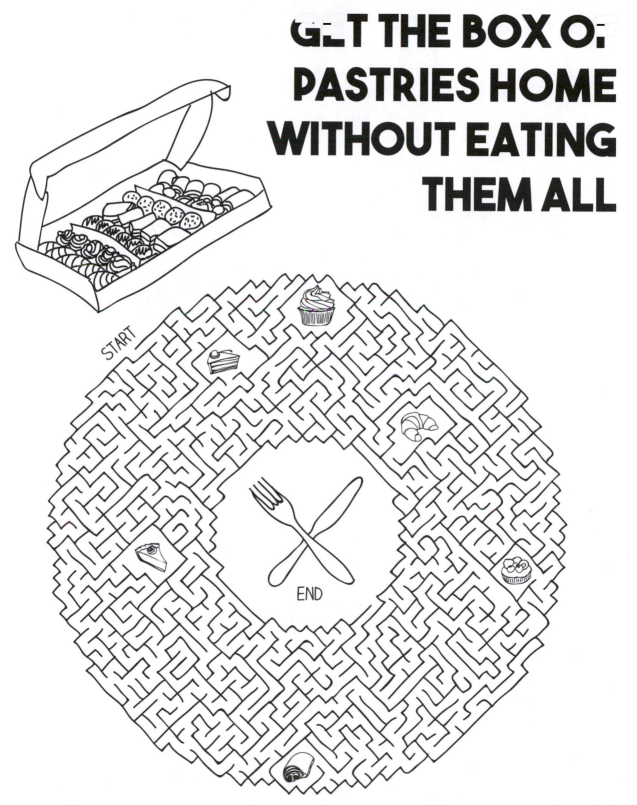

START

END

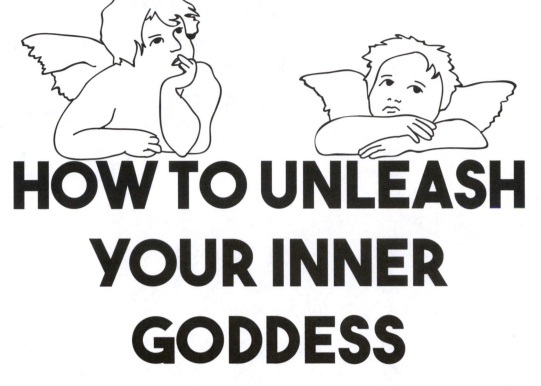

# HOW TO UNLEASH YOUR INNER GODDESS

Are you a hippie? That's cool. We all secretly wish we could be reincarnated as Kate Hudson in *Almost Famous* and capture the heart of a *Rolling Stone* reporter while touring the country with a rock band. (We downloaded a meditation app, used it once, and then watched *Almost Famous* in a sweatsuit while clipping our toenails and called it a day.) Whatever your Hippieness Authenticity Level may be, here are a few techniques for polishing up the old chakras.

1. Designate a space in your home that is just for you. Create an altar by hanging whimsical birth art and power selfies. Light a few dozen candles. Envision holding your baby in your arms. Maybe cradle a cantaloupe and rock it back and forth a bit.

2. Spend an evening making watercolor paintings of huge vaginas.

3. Play Gregorian chants or that ambient European electronica stuff that yoga teachers love.

4. Recite affirmations such as "I am a strong, powerful, birthing woman" or "It's okay to talk to yourself" while envisioning your future, which involves pushing a watermelon out of a pinhole and/or awake surgery.

5. Get one of those stones that says "Relax" and hold it for a while.

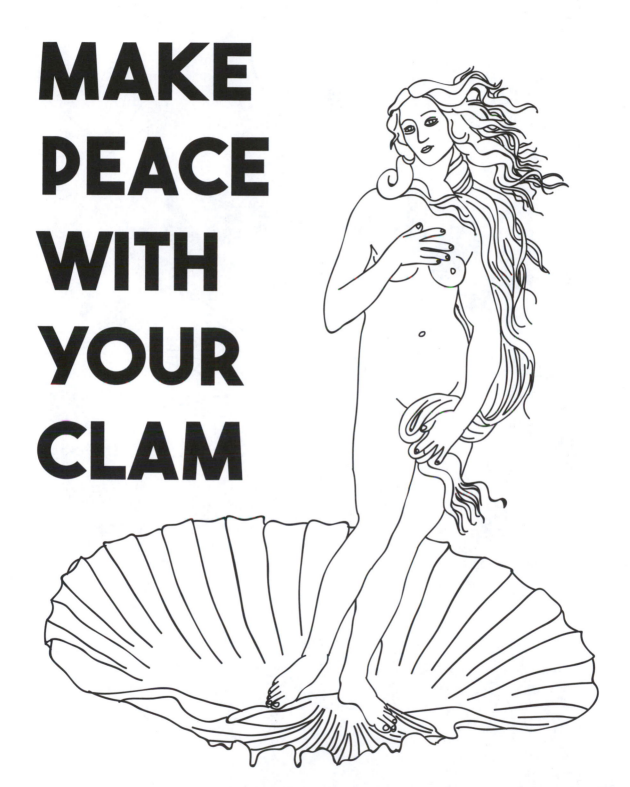

MAKE PEACE WITH YOUR CLAM

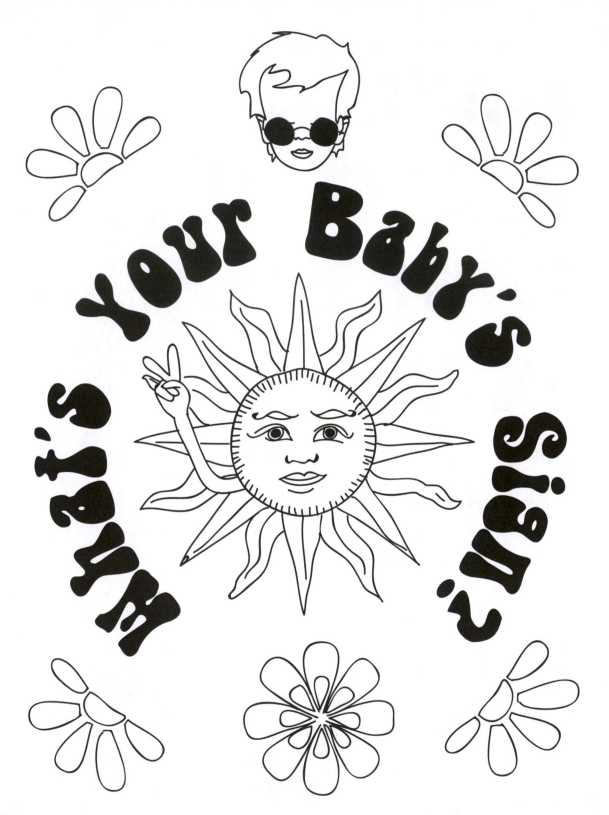

What's Your Baby's Sign?

Astrology is the ~~science~~ practice of using the positions of celestial objects to ~~reveal facts~~ guess about stuff that's going on down here on Planet Earth. Use your baby's star sign to reveal lots of secret information about what type of person he or she will be. Maybe.

My baby's due date is _____, so he/she is a _____.

GUIDE:

| | |
|---|---|
| ARIES | 21 MARCH-20 APRIL |
| TAURUS | 21 APRIL-21 MAY |
| GEMINI | 22 MAY-21 JUNE |
| CANCER | 22 JUNE-23 JULY |
| LEO | 24 JULY-23 AUGUST |
| VIRGO | 24 AUGUST-23 SEPTEMBER |
| LIBRA | 24 SEPTEMBER-23 OCTOBER |
| SCORPIO | 24 OCTOBER-22 NOVEMBER |
| SAGITTARIUS | 23 NOVEMBER-21 DECEMBER |
| CAPRICORN | 22 DECEMBER-20 JANUARY |
| AQUARIUS | 21 JANUARY-19 FEBRUARY |
| PISCES | 20 FEBRUARY-20 MARCH |

# Some divine secrets

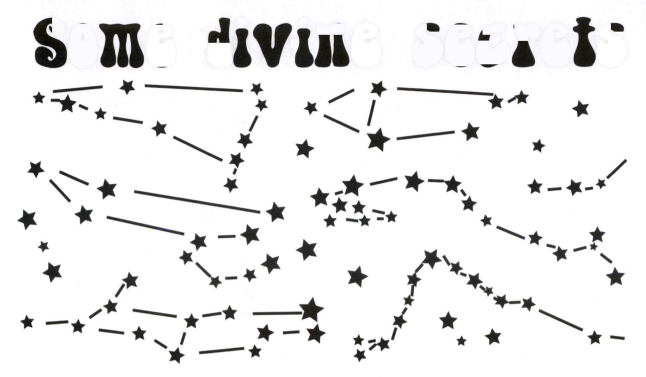

**Aries:** Aries babies are generally pissed off, much like Mars, their grandpa planet. Your baby will make an excellent politician, due to his or her tendency to yell and demand favors.

**Taurus:** Taurus babies love making quick decisions. In five years, you will not need to hem and haw about where you're going to eat dinner (it's going to be McDonald's, and it's going to be Right Now). They also love the opera, so play some *La Bohème* in the car while you eat your Happy Meals.

**Gemini:** This is the twin sign, which means your baby will have a split personality. He or she will be very "interesting," aka a huge pain in the ass. Your baby will probably be an artist and live at home until he or she is thirty-five.

**Cancer:** Cancers love things that are old. They also love garbage and refuse to throw away anything, including grandmothers, which is nice. They are very, very psychic. They can be dramatic at times, and love to emote. Invest in earplugs.

**Leo:** Leo babies are perfectionists who love to win. They demand the best of everything, including top-notch hotels and accommodations. Make sure your nursery décor is on point if you're having a Leo, or prepare to feel the wrath of the lion.

**Virgo:** Virgo babies are extremely clean and love discussing their innermost feelings and emotions. They're very adaptable to situations, such as "Mommy needs you to be quiet because *The Bachelorette* is on."

# about your baby:

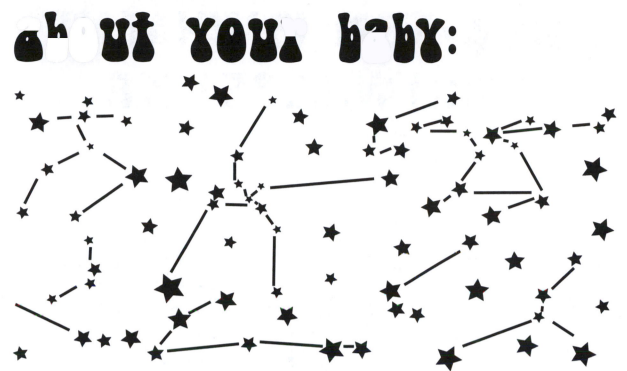

**Libra:** Libra babies are obsessed with being in love and can be selfish. They are also very beautiful and manipulative. Get ready to have all your money siphoned directly out of your checking account and into your baby's outstretched (but aesthetically pleasing) paws.

**Scorpio:** Scorpio babies notice everything and are extremely resourceful. They refuse to show weakness. Their resilience and eye for details make them very good lawyers. Law school is expensive, so start saving now.

**Sagittarius:** These babies love fast cars, unpredictability, and dancing at the clubs. If your baby is a girl, she will be a "horse person." If your baby is a boy, he will be very good at keg stands.

**Capricorn:** Capricorn babies are jealous and moody but also extremely charming. They will manipulate the pants off you, so be sure to stock up on extra pants.

**Aquarius:** These babies are very lovable but hard to know deeply. You will be enchanted by your Aquarius baby but will have difficulty pinning him or her down emotionally. This type of baby will be drawn toward alternative lifestyles, such as being a white person with dreadlocks or attending Lilith Fair.

**Pisces:** Pisces babies are psychic and make very good weatherpeople. They are extremely creative and good at all types of art, particularly oil painting and Shrinky Dinks.

# ...AND HERE IS WHAT MY BIRTH WILL BE LIKE

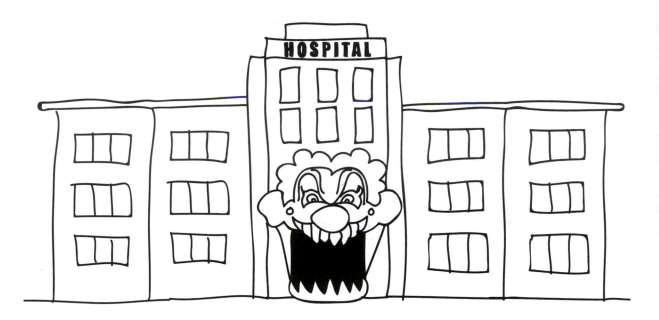

The Big Event is still months and months away, but even so, you're spending hours fantasizing about the magical, wondrous experience that awaits you. Or maybe you're just absolutely fucking terrified. Either way.

## Journal:

What I ~~think~~ hope will actually happen on the day I give birth:

_____
_____
_____
_____
_____
_____

*Hand this page over to a partner, who will prompt you for each blank, then read your epic creation out loud.*

When I think about giving birth, I just feel so _____ . Here's how
<sub>emotion</sub>
it's going to go. At _____ , my water is going to break. It'll look kind of like
<sub>time of day</sub>
_____ . I'll turn to _____ and say, "_____!"
<sub>liquid</sub> <sub>person</sub> <sub>exclamation</sub>
We'll get in the _____ and make our way to the _____ .
<sub>vehicle</sub> <sub>place</sub>
When we pull up, the nurse will say, "_____!" She'll give me
<sub>exclamation</sub>
some _____ and _____ , and lay me down on a nice big
<sub>food</sub> <sub>drink</sub>
_____ . I'll probably be in labor for _____ hours, so I'll have
<sub>piece of furniture</sub> <sub>number</sub>
to make sure to have lots of _____ . While I wait, maybe I'll get a chance to
<sub>noun</sub>
read a little _____ and watch _____ on the TV—you never
<sub>book</sub> <sub>TV show</sub>
know!

Then it'll be time to push. I'll want some music, so I'll tell _____ to put
<sub>person</sub>
on _____ . Once we really get going, I'll be saying, "_____!"
<sub>song</sub> <sub>exclamation</sub>
over and over. Finally I'll get to see your face and give you that _____ I
<sub>noun</sub>
made for you. The first thing you'll want to do is _____ . Maybe I'll give you a
<sub>verb</sub>
_____ to make you feel calm.
<sub>noun</sub>
That first night, we'll all get _____ hours of sleep and do lots of
<sub>number</sub>
_____ . Then we'll take you home in our _____ and show you
<sub>verb ending in -ing</sub> <sub>vehicle</sub>
your room, which will be decorated with _____ _____ .
<sub>color</sub> <sub>animal, plural</sub>
I think we'll call you _____ . I can't wait!
<sub>name</sub>

# YOU
# RIGHT
# NOW

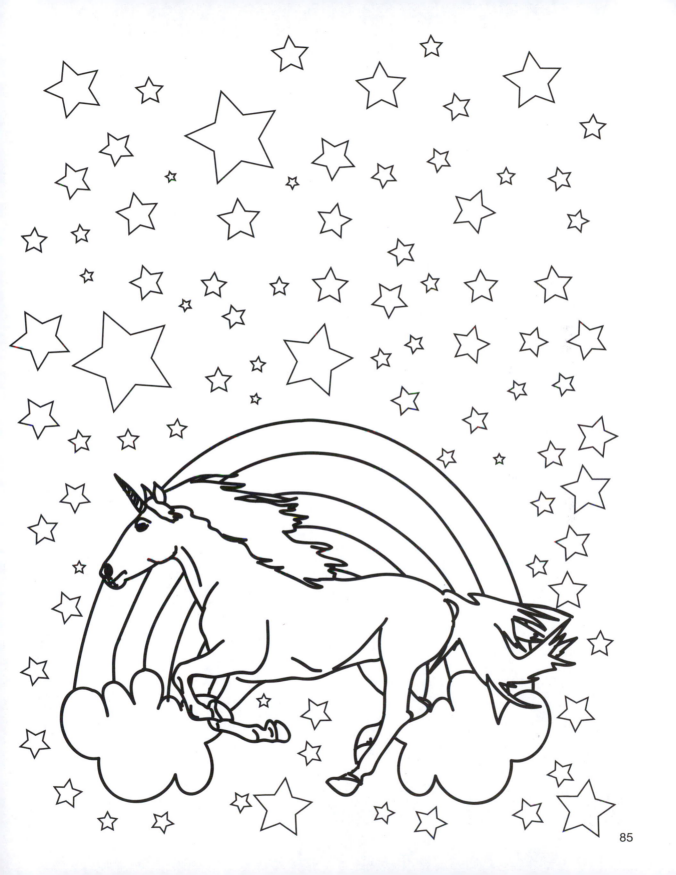

# GET
# IT
# OUT.

## THE THIRD TRIMESTER

# AT THE END

Have you ever heard the word "tetchy"?

It means sort of restlessly irritable, kind of like how dogs behave when there's a rainstorm on the way: scratching at walls, whining at windows, and generally acting crazy. It's the kind of word that you find yourself coming across in books from time to time, but never actually use, until that third trimester, when you become...yes...

Tetchy.

Except instead of scratching at walls (although that's completely acceptable behavior, too), you may find yourself doing things like bursting into tears for very literally no reason at all, washing every single piece of clothing in the house the second it becomes dirty, making insanely detailed lists, and pacing around the house while yelling about the air-conditioner settings. You can't sleep, and this makes you panic because you start thinking, "When this baby arrives I will never sleep again oh my god I need to sleep now," which is not exactly the most restful thought in the world. You make very attractive OOOOF sounds every time you roll over or have to get out of bed. Your acid reflux goes into overdrive. Weird crampy things start happening requiring anxious 4 a.m. Google searches. Strangest of all, you start behaving like an actual caged animal: walking in circles, moving things around for no discernible reason, and stacking and unstacking and restacking whatever's in front of you.

It all makes biological sense; it's called "nesting" (cute!), aka "frantically getting things in order in anticipation of bringing home a baby." When you're in the thick of it, though, you can know what's going on and still have zero control over what your mind and body are up to. It's funny, and it's crazy, and it mostly means that even if you don't feel "ready" for the baby to get here…guess what's about to happen?

What your body is telling you is that you *are* ready, and while your brain may be taking a second to catch up: You can totally do this. And you will sleep again (someday).


## Journal:

Completely inexplicable behavior that I do obsessively: _____.

Number of times I wake up every night: _____.

Loads of laundry I did this week: _____.

The last thing I googled: _____.

Panic level from 0–10*

0     1     2     3     4     5     6     7     8     9     10

*Don't panic.

# THINGS THAT WILL MAKE YOU CRY UNCONTROLLABLY

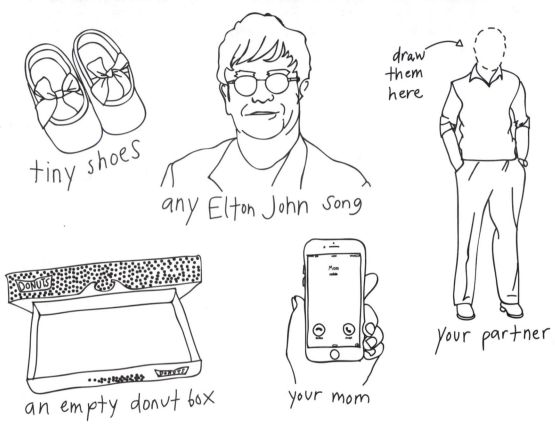

tiny shoes

any Elton John song

draw them here

your partner

an empty donut box

your mom

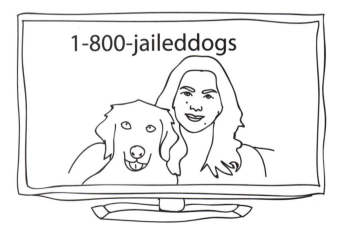

1-800-jaileddogs

that ASPCA commercial where Sarah McLachlan shows you a full minute of dogs in jail

# DISTRACT THYSELF

The end of pregnancy is very exciting and also sort of miserable. Having lots of stuff to distract yourself with helps.

Some suggestions:

☐ Bake at least ten banana breads and freeze them "for after the baby comes," with the full knowledge that they will be consumed by the end of the week.

☐ Make a birth playlist so that your partner can DJ your delivery, knowing that when it actually gets played, you will be busy giving birth and uninterested in hearing anything other than the words "Here is your baby."

☐ Exfoliate various body parts.

☐ Make a list of all the ways in which you are superior to your partner (including "gestated entire person" and "am just better, generally").

☐ Buy a box of Magic Erasers and use them to clean every single mark off every single one of your walls.

☐ Decide the couch looks better somewhere else. Enlist someone to help you move it. Decide it looked better where it used to be. Move it back.

☐ Count the coins in your spare change jar. Use them all to buy mini Snickers bars.

*Journal:*

Some more genius ways I've discovered to pretend that time is not moving at the speed of a football game:

_____

_____

# CIRCLE THE 3 THINGS THAT ARE CURRENTLY MAKING YOU THE MOST INSANE

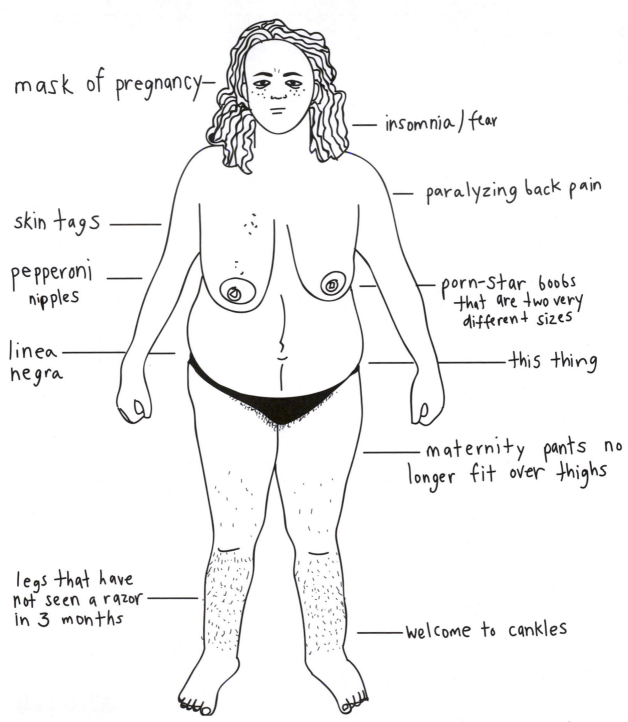

mask of pregnancy—

insomnia/fear

paralyzing back pain

skin tags —

pepperoni nipples

porn-star boobs that are two very different sizes

linea negra

this thing

maternity pants no longer fit over thighs

legs that have not seen a razor in 3 months

welcome to cankles

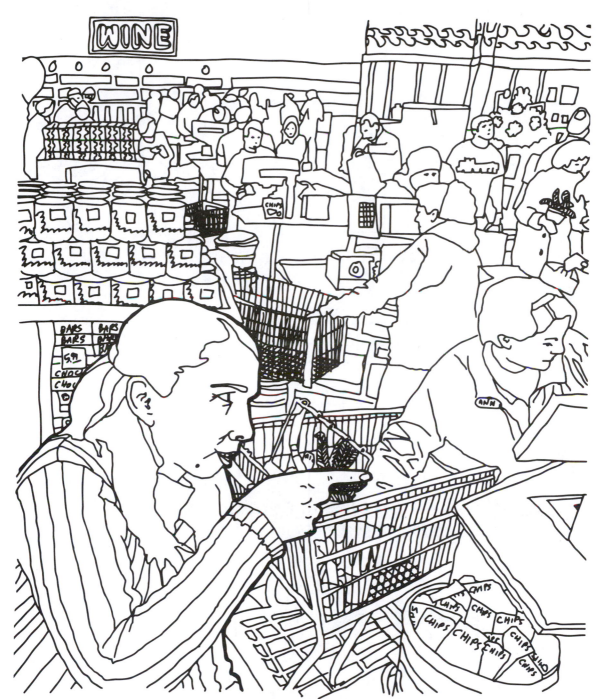

**DON'T YOU LOVE IT WHEN STRANGERS GIVE YOU PARENTING ADVICE?** Check here → ☐ No

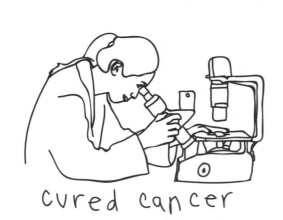

cured cancer

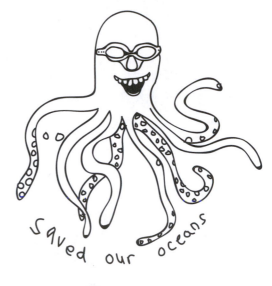

saved our oceans

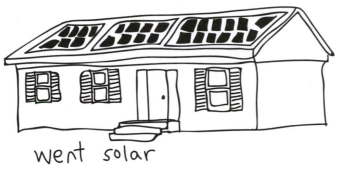

went solar

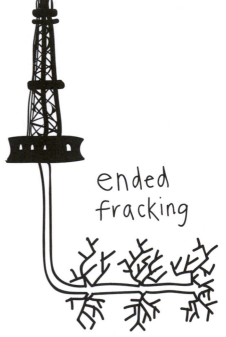

ended fracking

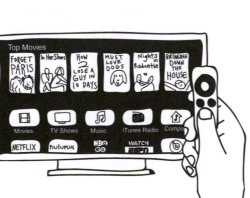

made apple TV work

# TOP FIVE

## WHAT FEATS HAVE YOU ACCOMPLISHED THUS FAR IN YOUR PREGNANCY?

1. _____
2. _____
3. _____
4. _____
5. _____

*Journal:*

**I deserve a medal for (*circle all that apply*):**
a) Still being able to walk (kind of)
b) Shaving my legs (once in a while)
c) Not buying a/n _____ [fill in the blank]
d) Growing an entire person
e) Permitting my partner to sleep in my bed (even though I'd rather it just be me and my lifeboat-size pillow)
f) Not eating every Ho Ho I wanted to eat (just most of them)
g) Being a moon goddess, basically

**I would like this medal to arrive in the form of:**
a) Extremely expensive jewelry
b) One of those heart-shaped cardboard boxes with cream-filled chocolates inside
c) Massages for days
d) Someone else taking over the actual birthing process, please
e) 12 straight hours of sleep
f) Hugs

# THINGS

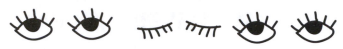

# THAT

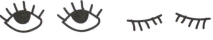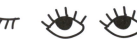

# MAKE

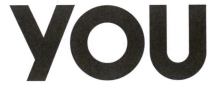

# YOU

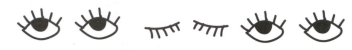

# TIRED

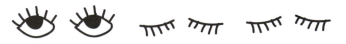

ACTIVITY BOOKS
BEING AWAKE
BLINKING YOUR EYES
BREATHING
CONVERSATION
DOCTOR APPOINTMENTS
EATING
EXERCISING
GROCERY SHOPPING
HEALTHY EATING
INSURANCE COMPANIES
MOVING
PEOPLE
PUTTING ON CLOTHING
PUTTING ON SHOES
SITTING
STANDING
THINKING
WALKING
WORK
YOUR DOGS
YOUR MOTHER
YOUR PARTNER

*Find the hidden words describing the many, many things in your life that are presently exhausting you to the point of tears. (Spoiler: It's everything. Mostly your mom.)*

```
E E P T X V K K E U Y I J A W E E I J X Q F C S J L F F D O
L E N C H U Z N V O P N C Y J R V G L W E O R C Z V F O C S
P E X G P E U B U V X S D R I V F X J P K G X N M X C Y O S
O E K L J K A R U M P U A C T I V I T Y B O O K S T P O N T
E T J A C E P L K T H R Y F B J S A O F E R O P O N W U V V
P M H V W A C P T Z H A E I D A R D E Q T H Y R X H W R E S
N H X I R A X H F H G N I K L A W P N O C V A M Y K X D R K
S Y M T N Q G K I C Y C O O M H L A Z I B P B L H F U O S X
J E N B L K W N G W L E V H G X B D J M P K W G E Q L G A R
H E Y J K M I N I F W C A W O R K J S O P V J H L U F S T V
R S K E D T I N C E I O R T M X Z V I G N V I Q U Y N I X
V M Z E R H A X G X B M D I I Y I N Q S E N V C A R J M O W
B O F C T U O X T A P P O S L N T J S D J I O Y W B F I N A
Z L Y A O L O F L Y B A M N H M G E J L F P Y R Z G V C P X
O Y E F W M F Y Q I C N L X E S O R X F C P E U S I J V B E
G R C T V Q G G G V N I G N I H T O L C N O G N I T T U P C
B O B N B T D N K N I E T T S F I L S N Z H X K Q I A T O X
O S H F E G G Q I O I S L N V B W X W G W S L N H S D Z S O
W N G M N O I K T T S K O C S I V H O M L Y L I U F Q M F H
L G U I B W G F V V A G N Q Q G Q E E L Y R Z C V O D S W C
V E V I I K U Q D C N E M I L N T I Q G Y E T T J Y J N O W
D O K L D Y P M J I P Z N A L M B G G N W C Q P C S I A O S
M S F H M H W P T G D Z G L P B C Y S I B O C W I J W N P E
V U Q Q T H M T K B Y D U B U I S F S S E R B L N D I H B K
E J M H A K U S C Q R V C T E I Z U L I K G P X Q S L I R Z
T K S H V P L X Z C O A P T T N U Q R C W O A S L A N C W F
O D O D F E T B M U Y J T T H Q X R J R B X C B K X I Z E J
R R W Y G N W N X M O E I N L P P P N E X M W X C T N V B C
G P Z V Y G F Y I B C N N B R C F Y E X F E N Q P Y S U L A
R E H T O M R U O Y G Y W C I I B P Y E S T A N D I N G I R
```

Tip: Ice cream never made anyone tired. Go eat some ice cream.

# 3 THINGS TO DO IN THE MIDDLE OF THE NIGHT WHEN YOU CAN'T SLEEP

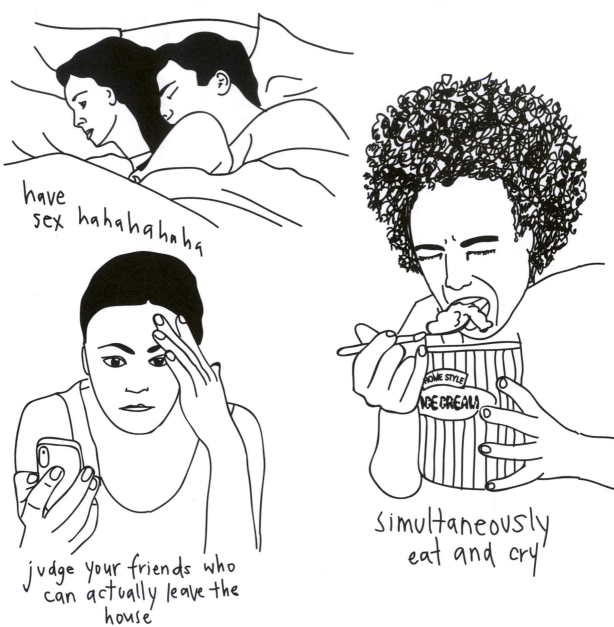

have sex hahahahaha

judge your friends who can actually leave the house

simultaneously eat and cry

# UNSCRAMBLE THE THINGS THAT WILL NEVER BE THE SAME ONCE YOU HAVE THIS BABY

1. **ACUSHYMOTOR**

\_ \_ \_ \_   \_ \_ \_ \_ \_ \_ \_

2. **OURGRIMYAREA**

\_ \_ \_ \_   \_ \_ \_ \_ \_ \_ \_ \_

3. **PELES**

\_ \_ \_ \_ \_

4. **ATEETHINGWIGINSTIL**

\_ \_ \_ \_ \_ \_ \_   \_ \_ \_ \_   \_ \_ \_ \_ \_ \_ \_

5. **NICETROUSER**

\_ \_ \_ \_ \_ \_ \_ \_ \_ \_ \_

6. **TEEREMIF**

\_ \_ \_ \_   \_ \_ \_ \_

7. **OLFACTORYROOFERUH**

\_ \_ \_   \_ \_ \_ \_ \_   \_ \_   \_ \_ \_ \_   \_ \_ \_

8. **AREHOYURT**

\_ \_ \_ \_   \_ \_ \_ \_ \_

# WHEN I HEAR THE WORD "STIRRUPS," I THINK...

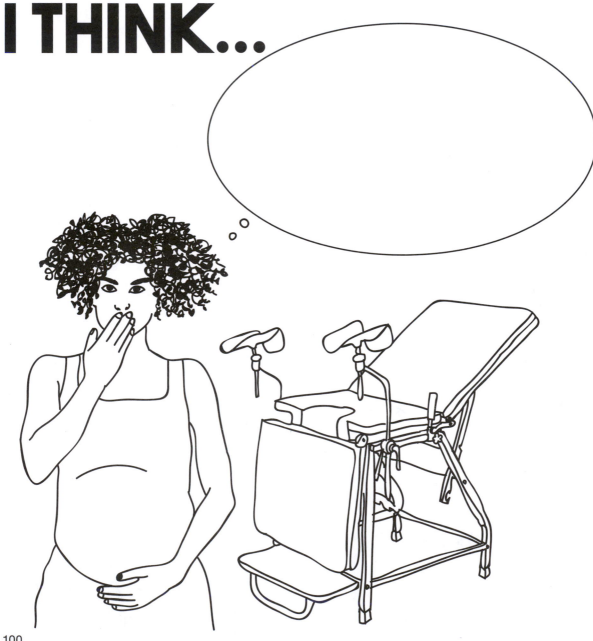

# THINGS STRANGERS SAY TO YOU

These are actual sentences that actual people appear to think are good things to say to pregnant women. Color in the ones you've heard in black until the words disappear. If you haven't heard them all yet, just wait: There's still time.

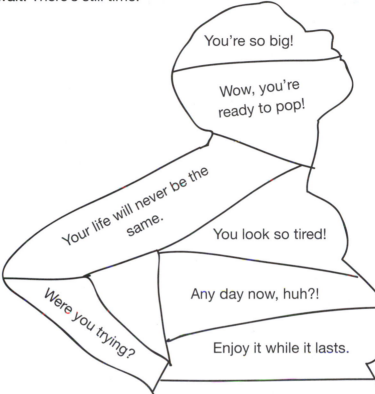

You're so big!

Wow, you're ready to pop!

Your life will never be the same.

You look so tired!

Were you trying?

Any day now, huh?!

Enjoy it while it lasts.

You should eat some crackers if you're feeling sick.

I can totally tell from the way you're carrying that you're having a boy/girl!

Are you sure there's just one in there?! Hahahaha.

You're STILL pregnant? Hahahaha.

Get in your sleep while you still can! HAAAAAA.

*Journal:*

I actually don't really mind when people tell me _____.

But if I could never hear this sentence again, that'd be supercool, thanks: _____
_____.

Here is what I secretly want to say to every single person who tells me I look like I'm "ready to pop": _____
_____.

# Quiz

Labor gets a bad rap. While it's not exactly a "relaxing" experience, the hours you spend bringing your child into the world—whether at home, at a hospital, or in a running stream while listening to birdcalls and slathering your body in organic coconut oil—will contain some of the most magical moments in your entire life. They also contain a lot of less-than-magical moments, and you will probably poop on the table (someone had to tell you).

*Find out how ready you are for the big show.*

1. Which of the following is not a sign that labor is beginning?
    a) Cramping, but not the "Oh dear I think I'm getting my period" kind; the worst kind
    b) Peeing becomes a part-time job
    c) Something called a "bloody show" happens, and the less we speak about this the better
    d) The baby "drops," which means you can breathe again

2. After you have the baby, the nurse will probably give you (*circle all that apply*):
    a) A bottle of champagne
    b) A mesh fishing net
    c) A box of maxi pads the size of life rafts
    d) Swaddling lessons

3. "Latching on" is:
    a) The part of labor where you put your feet in the stirrups
    b) The thing you do to your partner's hand during contractions
    c) Breastfeeding success
    d) One of the steps in the car-seat installation manual that I haven't read yet (but am totally planning to. Eventually)

4. Which of these items will not make labor more fun?
    a) Lip balm
    b) A pretty nightgown to wear instead of the hospital-issue gown
    c) Ice cubes
    d) A TV streaming *E! True Hollywood Story* 24/7

5. An epidural is:

a) A balloon-like contraption that your doctor may use to make you dilate more quickly and move labor along

b) An uncomfortably large, terrifying-looking needle that delivers drugs directly into your spinal cord

c) The part of delivery where your partner cuts through the cord and tries not to faint

d) The best

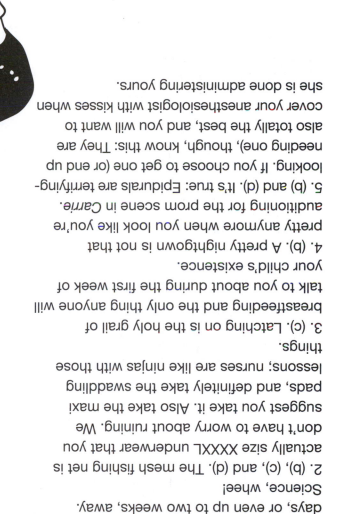

# answers

1. All of these can be can be signs that labor is beginning. Or that the baby is still several days, or even up to two weeks, away.

2. (b), (c), and (d). The mesh fishing net is actually size XXXXL underwear that you don't have to worry about ruining. We suggest you take it. Also take the maxi pads, and definitely take the swaddling lessons; nurses are like ninjas with those things.

3. (c). Latching on is the holy grail of breastfeeding and the only thing anyone will talk to you about during the first week of your child's existence.

4. (b). A pretty nightgown is not that pretty anymore when you look like you're auditioning for the prom scene in *Carrie*.

5. (b) and (d). It's true: Epidurals are terrifying-looking. If you choose to get one (or end up needing one), though, know this: They are also totally the best, and you will want to cover your anesthesiologist with kisses when she is done administering yours.

# THIRD TRIMESTER CHECK-IN

I am _____ weeks pregnant.

According to the Internet, my baby is the size of a/an _____.

This makes me feel _____.

I only want to wear _____.

The part/s of my body that is/are annoying me the most is/are my _____.

I really love my _____, though.

If I even think about _____, I want to throw up.

I still have to _____ before the baby gets here.

The best thing that happened this week was _____.

The worst thing that happened this week was _____.

When I think about my partner, the primary word that comes to mind is _____.

I really miss _____.

I'm so excited to _____.

The baby's movements remind me of _____.

Mostly I feel pretty _____.

I want to eat _____ RIGHT NOW.

# YOUR BABY'S DEVELOPMENT

**Week 26:** If you're having a boy, the parts of his body that he will spend the rest of his life scratching in inappropriate places have started to descend.

**Week 35:** Your baby's kidneys are fully developed, and he is peeing inside you. Aw.

**Week 39:** You are officially "full term" and probably pretty uncomfortable, thanks to the fact that your mammoth child is squishing your intestines up into your shoulders.

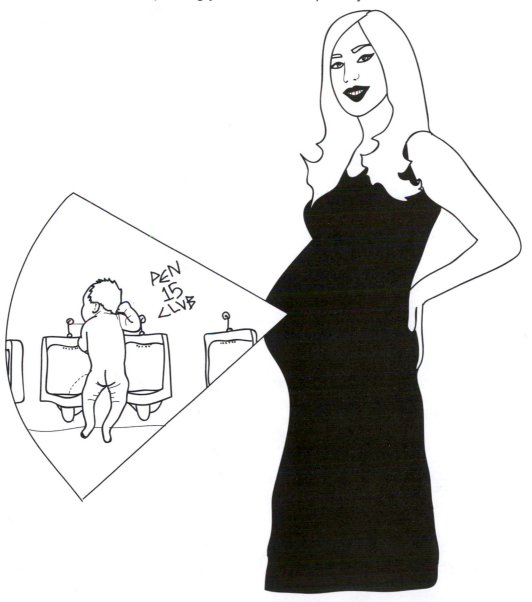

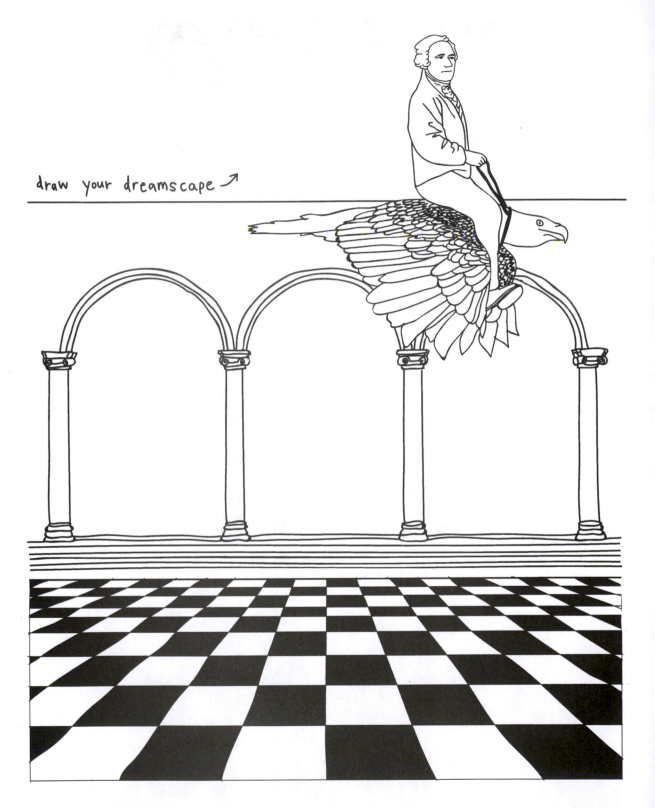

draw your dreamscape ↗

# TOP FIVE

## WHAT WERE YOUR FIVE CRAZIEST PREGNANCY DREAMS?

1. _____
2. _____
3. _____
4. _____
5. _____

## Journal:

**I have had the following "common pregnancy dreams" (*circle all that apply*):**

 a) A dream revealing my baby's gender
 b) A dream about an animal growing into a bigger animal
 c) A dream in which I took the baby out of my uterus and then put it back
 d) A dream about giving birth to an animal (this one: _____ )
 e) A dream about an ex-lover
 f) A dream in which I was submerged in a body of water
 g) An "I forgot the baby" dream
 h) A dream about giving birth to an inanimate object (this one: _____ )
 i) A dream about that thing from *Alien*

**Tonight, I'd really like to dream about:** _____.

# CIRCLE THE OBJECTS THAT ARE MOST IMPORTANT TO YOU RIGHT NOW

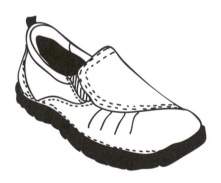

hideous but comfortable footwear

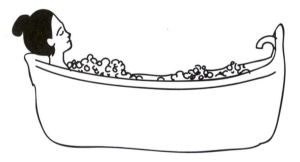

bubble baths

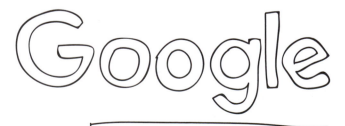

Google

everything|

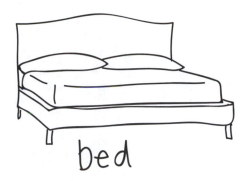

bed

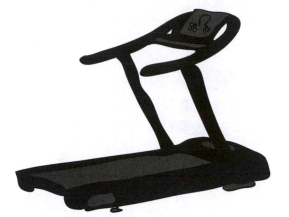

exercise

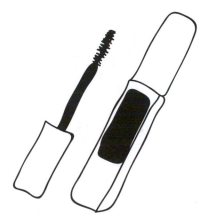

Waterproof
mascara

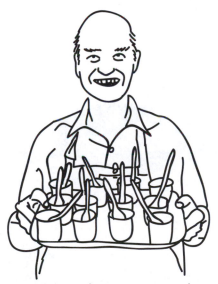

Costco Samples

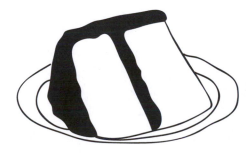

caaaaake

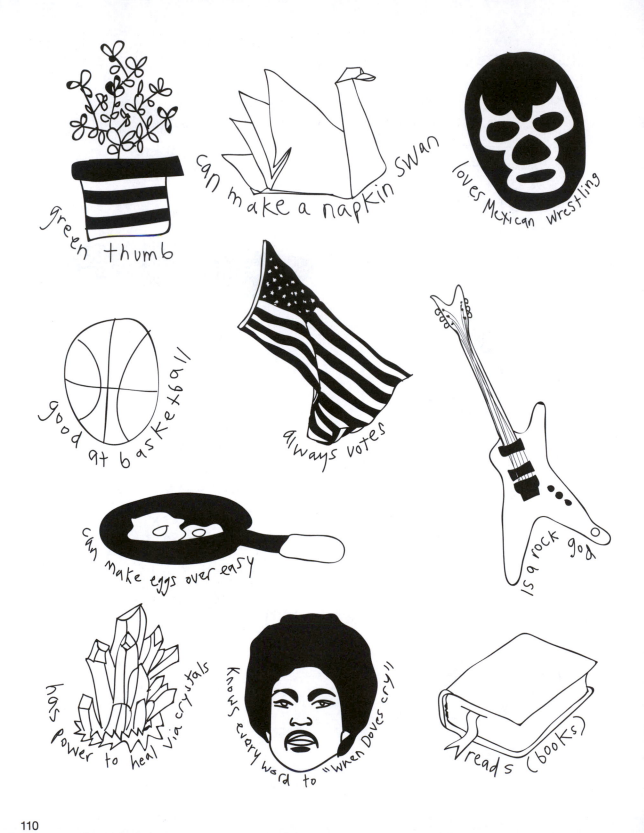

green thumb

can make a napkin swan

loves Mexican wrestling

good at basketball

always votes

is a rock god

can make eggs over easy

has power to heal via crystals

knows every word to "when Doves cry"

reads (books)

# 3 QUALITIES YOU HOPE THE BABY GETS FROM YOU, AND 3 QUALITIES YOU HOPE THEY GET FROM YOUR PARTNER

## FROM YOU:

1. _____

2. _____

3. _____

## FROM YOUR PARTNER:

1. _____

2. _____

3. _____

# WHAT TO BRING WITH YOU TO THE HOSPITAL

There is no shortage of parenting websites and books dispensing endless tips on what you should bring to the hospital when it's go time. You've probably already stocked up on flip-flops (because gross hospital floors), going-home outfits for yourself and the baby, and easy-reading magazines. You're good on miniature toiletries and cozy socks. But there are a few more necessities that many lists neglect.

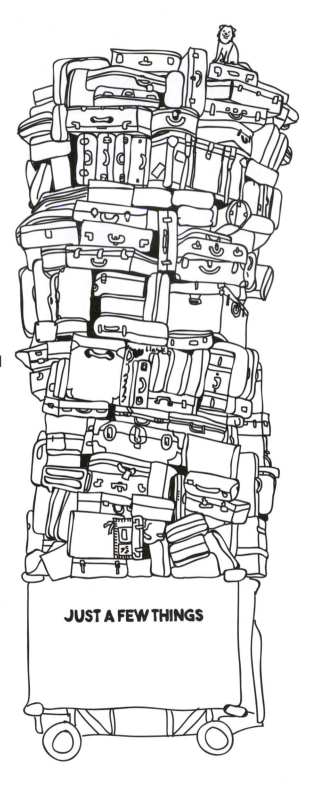

JUST A FEW THINGS

## 1. Dark-Colored Everything

Is something going to touch your body? Cool. It better be black. We can go into specifics, but let's just say "maxi pad that, despite its disturbing size, will not be especially effective in containing the volume of fluids emitted from your person," and leave it at that.

## 2. Ear Plugs

Hospitals are not quiet places. And even if you're so exhausted post-birth that you feel like you could snore through a St. Patrick's Day parade, you may not get a private room, and you may not be *quite* tired enough to ignore the fact that your roommate apparently has twenty-five people in her immediate family, and all of them feel the need to celebrate. Loudly.

## 3. A Pillow for Your Partner

As much as you might feel like the other adult involved in this situation should suffer with you a little (they may be tired, too, but they are not simultaneously leaking milk and other fluids from their body in epic quantities while trying to figure out what the hell this whole "latching on" business is about), hospital benches really do suck to sleep on. Throw the guy or gal a bone.

## 4. An Advocate

You may already know how you want your birth to go. You may be comfortable being pretty damn clear about those desires. But it does happen, from time to time, that things like pain cause people to do stuff like be unable to communicate anything at all, up to and including answers to important medical decisions. Have someone whom you trust present (whether your partner, a close friend or relative, or a doula), and make sure they're willing and able to speak on your behalf if you're not up to the task yourself.

---

### A Brief Note on Doulas

If labor is like climbing Mt. Kilimanjaro, doulas are like Sherpas. They are there for you through pregnancy, labor, and the postpartum period. They help you advocate for yourself and provide you with physical and emotional support. They've seen it all, and they can be a hugely reassuring presence in a moment of great need. If you can afford it, you might also want to consider hiring a doula to help you with the rest of your life, forever and ever, from holding your hand during root canals to tucking you in at night (with lavender oil, obviously). Because for real: Doulas are the best.

---

# PLEASE, LEAVE THESE AT HOME

**1. Any Item of Clothing That You Really Like, or That Would Make You Cry Were It to Be Ruined**
It will probably be ruined.

**2. Books**
Sorry, this is not happening. Think *Star* magazine, not *War and Peace.*

**3. Pants in Your Former Size**
Sorry again, but this is also not happening (not for a while, at least). Bring along a pair from when you were six months pregnant.

**4. Expectations**
The birth experience is nothing if not completely and utterly unpredictable. It will very likely not go how you expect it to go. But that's okay, because it will also be extraordinary and exciting and remarkable and *yours.*

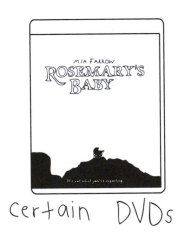

certain DVDs

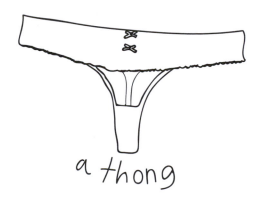

a thong

| | | | | | | | | | | | | | | | | | | | | | | | | | | | | |
|Britannica|Britannica|Britannica|Britannica|Britannica|Britannica|Britannica|Britannica|Britannica|Britannica|Britannica|Britannica|Britannica|Britannica|Britannica|Britannica|Britannica|Britannica|Britannica|Britannica|Britannica|Britannica|Britannica|Britannica|Britannica|Britannica|Britannica|Britannica|Britannica|
|1|2|3|4|5|6|7|8|9|10|11|12|13|14|15|16|17|18|19|20|21|22|23|24|25|26|27|28|29|

those books you've been meaning to read

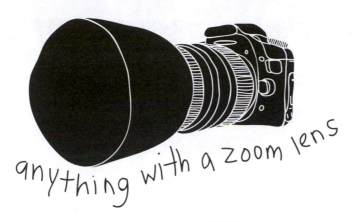

anything with a zoom lens

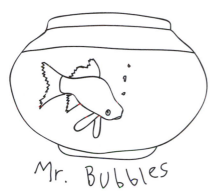

Mr. Bubbles

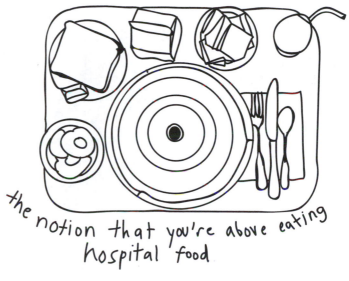

the notion that you're above eating
hospital food

dear self,
    please, for the love of god, do not forget
to bring these things with you to the
    hospital:

1. _____

2. _____

3. _____

4. _____

5. _____

# TOP FIVE

## WHAT ARE YOUR MOST HORRIFYING PREGNANCY CRAVINGS?

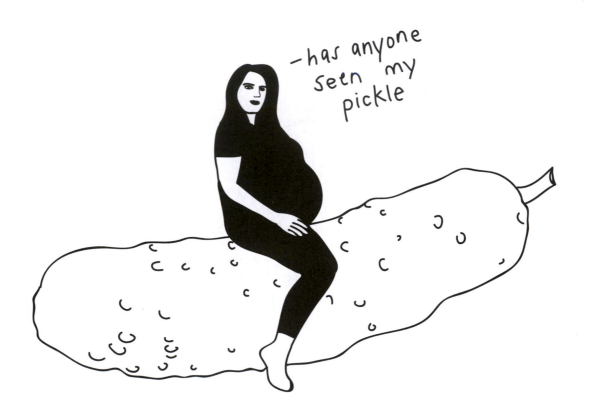

1. _____

2. _____

3. _____

4. _____

5. _____

# EAT ME

1. Draw a line between each craving and the topping you would like to put on it. Matching one food to multiple toppings or matching one topping to multiple foods is strongly encouraged.

2. Cross out any foods or toppings that you can't even think about without gagging.

3. Put stars next to any foods or toppings that you could literally eat your weight in right now.

| | |
|---|---|
| Pizza | Hot Sauce |
| Bagel | Butter |
| Ice Cream | Cheese |
| Peanut Butter Sandwich | Chocolate Anything |
| Chinese Food | Banana |
| Steak | Ketchup |
| Mashed Potatoes | Soy Sauce |
| Hamburger | Tomato Sauce |
| White Rice | Cheese Whiz |
| Brownies | Cool Whip |
| Pickles | Frosting |
| French Fries | Pepperoni |
| Pasta | Mustard |
| Cake | Salt |
| Fruit | Ranch Dressing |
| Chocolate Anything | Vinegar |

Draw one thing you've never wanted to eat before but now desire with the heat of a thousand suns

One thing you've always loved and now can hardly stand to look at, which sucks:

_____

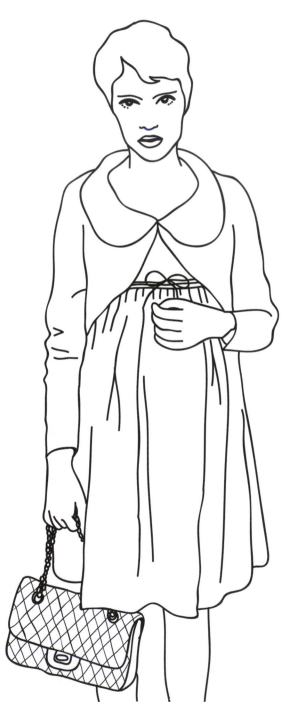

# THE IMPATIENT WOMAN'S SUMMARY OF GOOGLEABLE INFORMATION ON EARLY LABOR SIGNS

We've all been there. You're late in your third trimester, and you desperately want to meet the little nugget who shares half your DNA and won't stop kicking you in the ribs. And so every time you feel a cramp, wiggle, or jiggle you ask yourself, "Was that something?!" You run to the bathroom to check your giant underthings for gross stuff. You can recite the dictionary definition of "Braxton Hicks." You don't even need to have your doctor on speed dial, because his phone number (and extension, and the number that you're "only supposed to call in case of an actual emergency") have been burned into your long-term memory.

You will google; it's inevitable. We don't care how strong you think you are against its deep, dark powers. Here's what you will find when you succumb to Google's clutches:

1. If you're between 38–42 weeks pregnant, you will probably go into labor soon.

2. Your water may break before active labor, but it probably won't.

3. You may or may not noticeably discharge something attractively called a "mucous plug" or a "bloody show" into your large lady underpants. This may mean that labor is coming in the next twenty-four hours, but it could also mean that it's weeks away.

4. An internal exam can reveal how far along you're dilated and effaced, but the information will be entirely unhelpful in terms of predicting when you'll go into labor.

5. You will almost surely not give birth on your due date, so don't expect to (unless you're having a scheduled C-section). About fifty percent of women give birth before their due date. The other fifty percent give birth after.

6. Your baby may or may not "drop" days, weeks, or hours before you go into labor. This does not help to predict the timeline but does help you breathe again. You can use all that air to help lug yourself to the bathroom, because you'll have to pee every five minutes.

7. If you have diarrhea, nausea, an achy pelvis, insomnia, and/or painful Braxton Hicks contractions while walking around Costco, congratulations, you are pregnant. At some point, you will likely give birth.

Your chances of discovering a buried prophetic GeoCities deep in the trenches of an anonymous What to Expect forum that tells you the exact date and time your bundle will make his or her appearance are slim to none (we know, we've looked).

Maybe take up knitting?

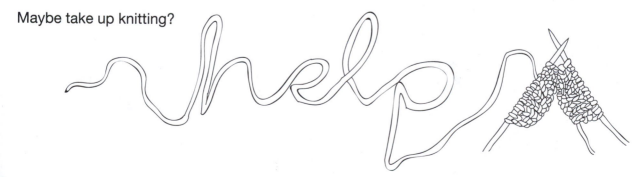

# HOW MANY STRANGERS HAVE CARESSED YOU TODAY?

this many

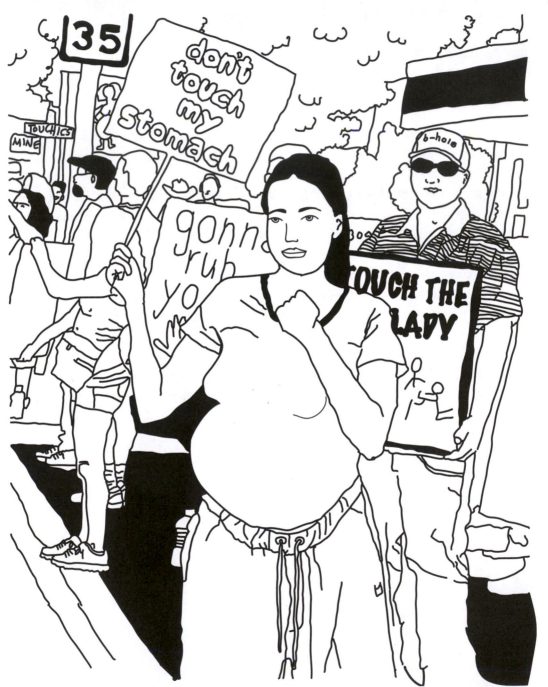

# THE PREGNANCY MEMORY BOX

The Pregnancy Memory Box is a thing we made up, a theoretical container for all your pregnancy memories and dreams. Here are a few things you might keep inside:

1. Brick of cheese eaten every afternoon at 3 p.m. because you "needed calcium."

2. "Ethereal, glowy" pregnancy photos in which you look neither ethereal nor glowy.

3. Hoop earrings (might as well say goodbye now, because they're not going on again until your child is at least three).

4. Rubber band for holding pants together.

5. Tweezers to remove random hormone-driven facial hairs (beards are in, right?).

6. Prenatal yoga DVD by the lady married to Alec Baldwin (unopened).

7. Sonogram picture of the first time you saw your baby and then ugly-cried for a full hour because you never knew how much you could love a tadpole.

Your own additions, please:

_____

_____

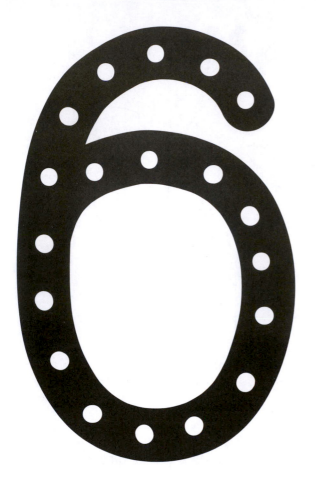 # **THINGS YOU CAN TRY TO GET THIS BABY OUT**

Somewhere around Week 39, you will start to really, really (really) want to get this show on the road. And if you pass The Great and Terrible Due Date without the arrival in your life of a whole bunch of tiny fingers and toes, it is very likely that desperation will set in, and it will set in hard.

Fortunately, there are tons and tons of things that you can try to get your baby out. And even though it is highly unlikely that any of them will actually result in a child being emitted from your person (despite the fact that the lady at the yarn store is 100 percent positive that it was the Kung Pao Chicken that did it for her daughter), hey: At least you've got something to do now besides call your doctor or midwife every five seconds—although obviously you're going to keep doing that, too.

## 1. **Eat Pineapple**
Pineapple apparently contains enzymes that help to "ripen the cervix." Unfortunately, said enzyme is only present in fresh pineapple (not canned). Fortunately, if you live in a tropical region, you are super in luck and will probably be able to sneeze out your baby.

## 2. Drink Womanly Teas

Certain herbal teas are said to stimulate uterine contractions. They are also usually rather unpleasant tasting and thus best ingested alongside a nice scone and some clotted cream. Consuming raspberry tea leaves will not make you happy, but the scone may be sufficient compensation.

## 3. Eat Spicy Foods

Nearly every article on the Internet about the practice of eating spicy foods to induce labor begins with the words "So there's no actual evidence that this works, but…" Which seems like a pretty solid vote of confidence. Spicy foods will not, in fact, kick off the birthing process, but they may give you a nice case of heartburn, so if your end goal is pain, and you don't really care whether it's coming from your uterus or your esophagus: ta daaaa!

## 4. Have Huge-Pregnant-Lady Sex

What's great about this one is that what theoretically functions to induce labor is the part where you have an orgasm. What's less great about this one is that there are few things on the planet less sexy and less likely to result in an orgasm than someone desperately trying to stimulate a clitoris that he or she is having serious trouble locating (see: huge pregnant lady).

## 5. Make a Labor Pizza

According to urban legend, there is a type of pizza that will immediately cause a woman to go into labor through the sheer volume of meat ingested. The ingredients include (but are of course not limited to) shredded mozzarella cheese, salami, pepperoni, ham, mushrooms, green peppers, extra onions, black olives, green olives, ground sausage, linguica, ground beef, whole garlic cloves, oregano, and parmesan cheese.

Labor pizza obviously does not work, but is a good excuse to eat pizza.

## 6. Stimulate Your Nipples While Bouncing on a Birthing Ball with Your Dog Sitting in a Corner Staring at You in Utter Confusion

Just do this because it's funny. (Maybe get it on videotape.)

P.S. If you just so happen to have your water break moments after drinking crappy tea/ingesting a few jalapeños/having an orgasm and are dead convinced that this was the result of your labor-inducing genius rather than a neat coincidence, congratulations! You, too, now get to join the annals of women whose stories, passed down through the ages, will result in generations of frantic nipple squeezers.

*List the things you tried to get the baby out of your body, and don't forget to note whether or not they worked! (If they did, maybe don't worry about checking off lists in activity books and go to the hospital instead.)*

## THING I TRIED

## WORKED    DID NOT WORK

top this labor pizza

# DON'T HAVE THE BABY IN THE CAR

AVOID A PANICKING PARTNER! TRAFFIC CONES! RED LIGHTS! FIND YOUR METICULOUSLY PACKED BAG THAT'S DISAPPEARED! WHY THE #$*& WON'T THE MAPS APP LOAD?!

START!

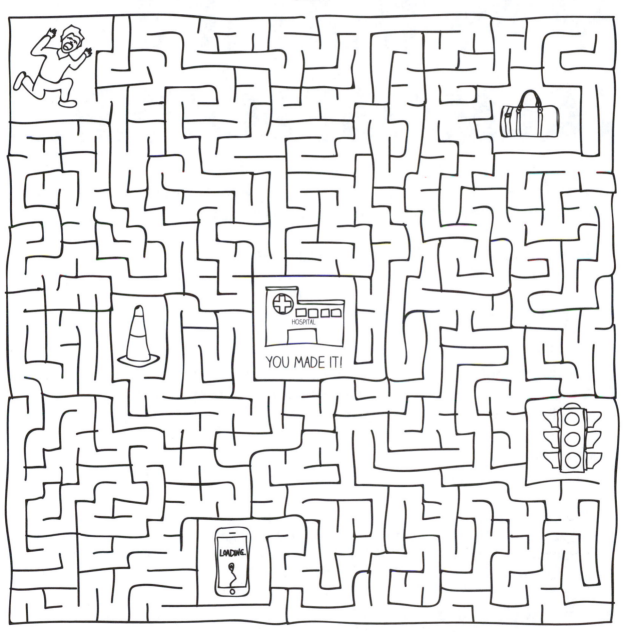

YOU MADE IT!

# NOW THAT IT'S (ALMOST) OVER...

Remember that day, several lifetimes ago, when you peed on a stick and your life changed forever? Wasn't it cute how little you knew then and how (relatively) much you know now?

*Go ahead: Write your former self a letter, and feel free to brag about how far you've come.*

Dear Nine-Months-Ago Me,

At this moment, I am _____ days from giving birth (according to my doctor. I am aware that the chances I will have a vaginal birth on the day that I am expected to are akin to the chances that I am gestating an Oompa-Loompa).

I gained _____ pounds, most of which was from:
   a) Pizza
   b) Tacos
   c) Cake
   d) Pizza, tacos, cake, stale bread, old cereal, and pretty much anything not nailed down
   e) Healthy whole foods like broccoli and squash, which I consumed while simultaneously polishing my halo

I cried at work _____ times (a day).

My partner is very lucky I only mentioned divorce _____ times.

I prepared for this baby by (*circle all that apply*):

    a) Taking birth classes

    b) Reading books

    c) Talking to friends who have kids

    d) Actually listening to my mother for the first time in my life

    e) Reading mommy blogs and swearing that when the day comes, I will make my preschooler bento-box lunches with sandwiches cut into the shapes of anime characters

    f) Watching Netflix and eating

    g) Chanting, meditating, drinking ionized tonics, and rubbing essential oils on my various chakras

    h) Designing and executing the perfect chevron nursery, one that is both tasteful and elegant

    i) Running a marathon, maintaining a vegan, gluten-free diet, doing yoga four times a day, and having lots of hot sex while also modeling for Victoria's Secret in my spare time because I am Gisele

When I first found out I was pregnant, I had no idea that I would soon discover: _____

_____

_____

_____

_____.

My favorite thing about this pregnancy was: _____

_____

_____

_____

_____.

I definitely could have lived without:_____

_____

_____

_____

_____.

The coolest thing I learned from this whole experience was: _____

_____

_____

_____

_____.

I still don't know how to _____
(but that's okay; that's what the Internet is for).

Now that it's almost over, I'm just so excited that: _____

_____

_____

_____

_____.

I wish I could go back in time and tell you: _____

_____

_____

_____

_____.

Let's go meet our baby.

Love,
Three-seconds-from-Becoming-a-Mama Me

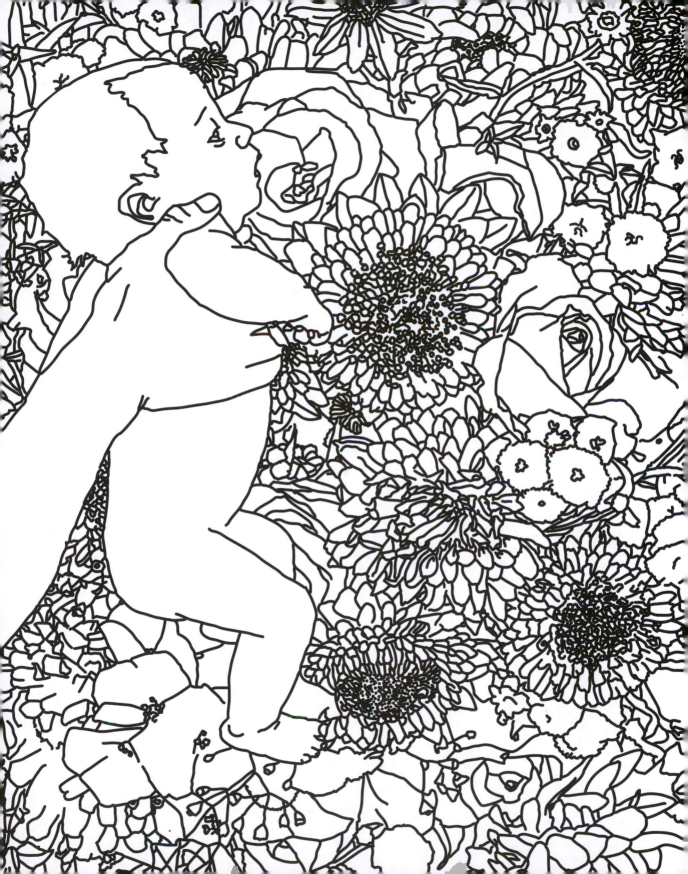

# WHAT
# IS
# SLEEP

# THE FOURTH TRIMESTER

# YOU ARE AMAZING (AND YOU CAN DO THIS)

So, you had a baby. You spent almost a year transforming a speck of sand into a human, and then—with all your tremendous female superpowers—you opened up your body, and a tiny, messy person emerged, beautiful and probably confused as to why it was so cold out in the world. You held your perfect baby, did a weird laugh-cry thing for hours, and in a single moment finally understood what true love is.

And now you're home and in the thick of one of the most challenging situations of your entire life.

Do you know what militaries do to get POWs to talk? They deprive them of sleep. As of the day of your child's birth, you have become a hostage, and your baby's job is to convey in no uncertain terms that while you may have been the center of the universe before, you have been usurped. It's an enormous adjustment, but all the fears and doubts you have are totally normal.

You might be worried that you are not cut out for this. That you'll be too tired to hold the baby after yet another sleepless night. That your partner isn't doing it right, or that he or she is doing it better than you (which, hello, is not allowed). That you won't know how to breastfeed. That your mother-in-law will never, ever go back home—or, worse, that she will, and you'll be left all on your lonesome to do this "parenting" thing.

Every mother has these worries. It's normal to be in love with your baby and simultaneously completely overwhelmed by your baby. It's also normal to sometimes just want your baby to go to sleep so you can play Candy Crush.

In short: Whatever you feel about this time in your life, it's okay. You are okay. You are in the middle of a massive life upheaval, so remember to take care of yourself. Eat something. Rest a little when you can. Forgive yourself. Ask for help if you need it, whether that means talking to a therapist or paying someone to do your laundry. Ask for meals. Ask for time to sleep. Ask for people to come over, or ask for them to leave.

You are a mom now. You're doing the best you can, and "your best" is everything it needs to be.

# REPEAT THESE AFFIRMATIONS

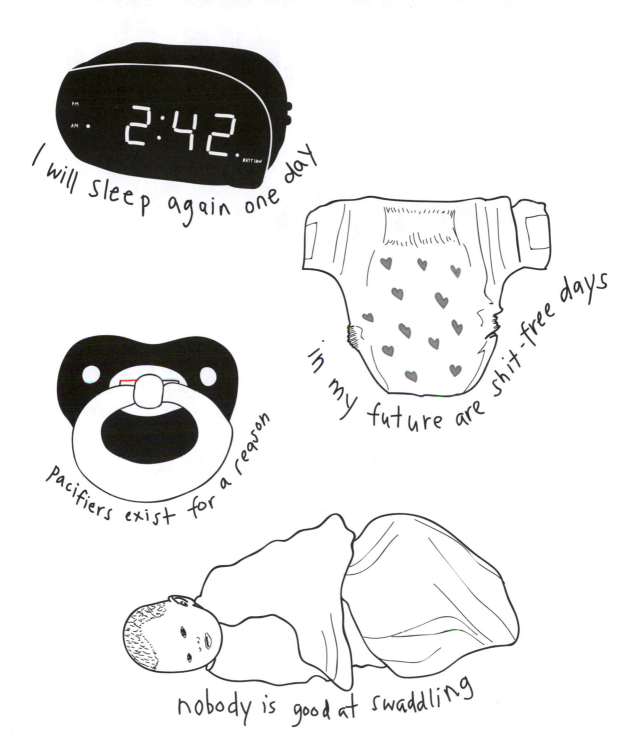

I will sleep again one day

Pacifiers exist for a reason

in my future are shit-free days

nobody is good at swaddling

# REAL HEROES ASK FOR HELP

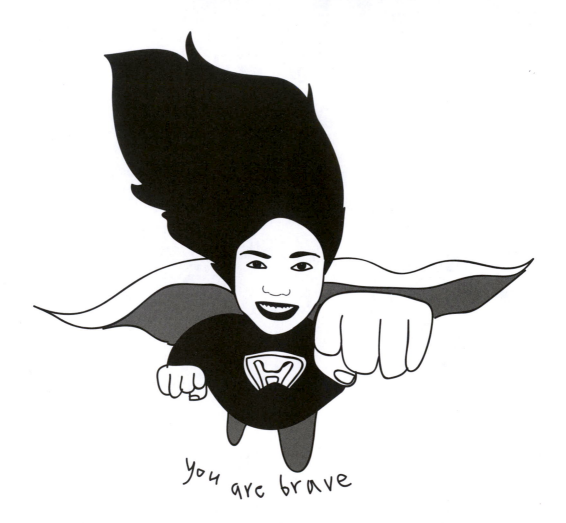

you are brave

Doctors, nurses, midwives, doulas, psychiatrists, and counselors can all be an important part of your support network. Asking for help is the bravest thing you can do.

# POSTPARTUM PAPER DOLL

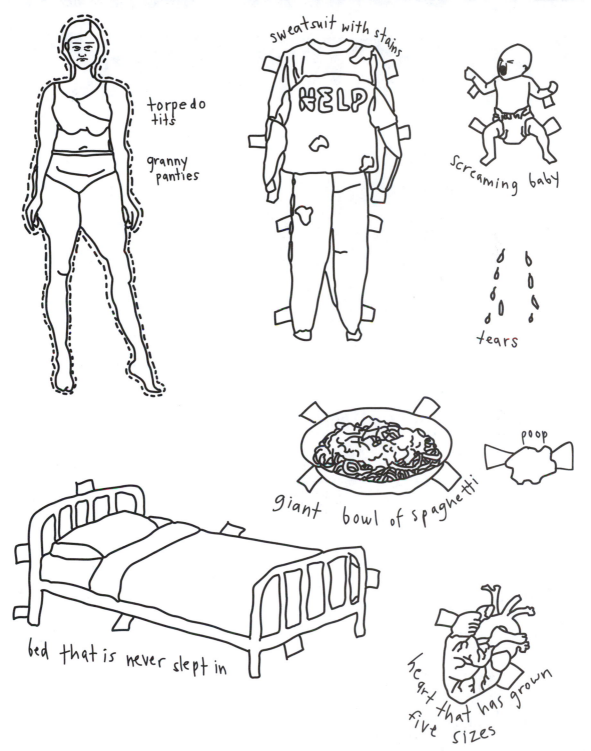

torpedo tits

granny panties

sweatsuit with stains

HELP

screaming baby

tears

giant bowl of spaghetti

poop

bed that is never slept in

heart that has grown five sizes

# NEWBORN PHOTOS:
# THE CLASSICS

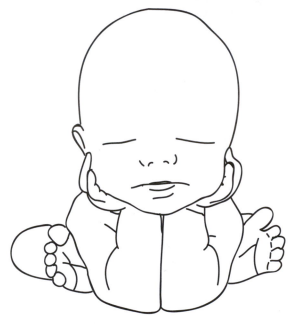

There are many unforgettable
moments in your child's life that you will forget because you
are sleep-deprived, but also because you are the most horrible
parent on Planet Earth according to several Internet articles.
Snapping regular photos of your adorable baby in various poses
and then Photoshopping them to look tan is the only way to
properly capture these amazing memories. Here's a list of
required Kodak moments.

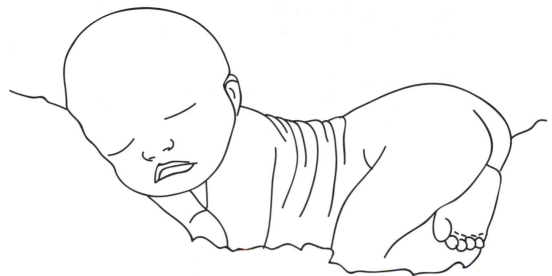

## 1. The Newborn Photo

Your baby looks like a constipated shar-pei, so you'll want to capture that. To optimize the beauty of this moment, place a faux fur vest from Forever 21 in an egg chair. Lay your sleeping baby on top, carefully folding her arms underneath her chin in a thoughtful, Rodin-esque pose.

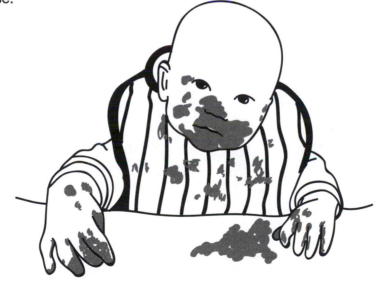

## 2. The "Here Is My Baby Covered in Disgusting Food" Photo

Your baby probably loves vegetables, whole grains that do not have gluten, probiotics, omega-3 fatty acids, and local, seasonal fruits (what a genius!). Or maybe he consumed those things for two weeks, after which you discovered the glorious ease of "pouches." Either way, it is literally impossible to make it through the first year of your baby's life without posting a photo of him or her covered in disgusting food to the Internet. Just try.

### 3. The Monthly Photo of Your Baby Wearing a Sticker

These stickers will enable you to save precious time by no longer having to use words to tell people how old your baby is. By placing a giant sticker on his chest, you can announce proudly to all the people who are dying to know that he is EIGHT MONTHS. You can use the time you save in not saying how old your baby is to knit tiny organic socks out of orphan alpaca hairs, or watch TV.

### 4. The Seasonal Photo of Your Baby Shoved into a Pumpkin

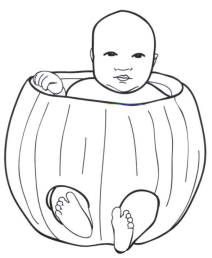

Is it Halloween? Do you have a baby? Achieve uproarious seasonal bliss by stuffing your spawn into a hollowed-out pumpkin. The monthlong reprieve between the pumpkin incident and the one where you settle your baby into a nest of electric holiday lights and itchy tinsel in nothing but a Santa hat will be enough to ensure no long-term psychological damage. This is how memories are made, people.

### 5. The Photo of Your Baby Wearing a Hilarious Graphic Onesie

Is your two-month-old a "ladies man"? Is your baby girl a "diva just like her mama"? Is your baby's "brother from another mother" a pug wearing sunglasses and a bow tie? If the answer to those questions is "Yes, absolutely," great. You will find no shortage of baby-enrobing options on the Internet. If the answer is "Oh my god NO," then sorry: People are going to buy you these things anyway. And will then demand that you take photographs of your baby wearing them and post them on Facebook.

I'M AN ALCOHOLIC BUT FOR MILK

# DRAW HAIR ON THE POSTPARTUM BALDING LADY

*All your awesome pregnancy hair fell out. It's super sad. Give yourself a brand-new do, and remember, that frizzy little regrowth halo won't last forever.*

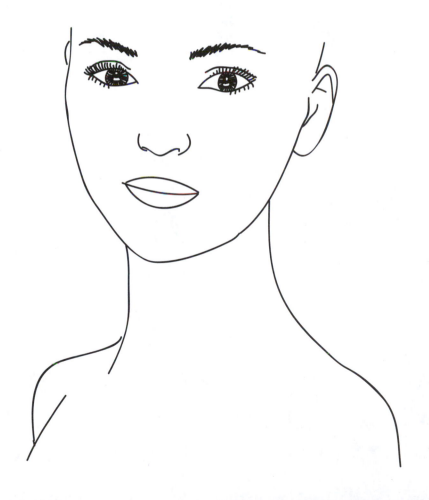

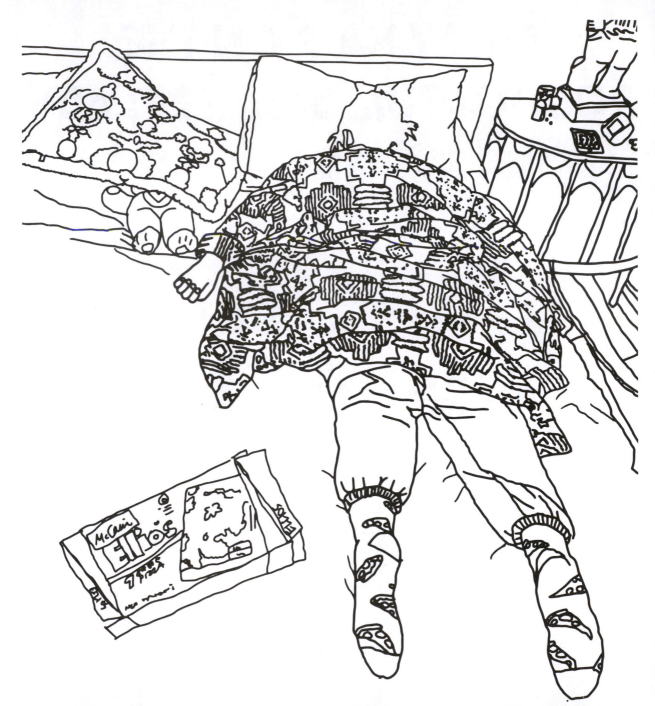

# SEXY DATE NIGHT

**LEAVE THE PIZZA. DON'T TOUCH ME ON YOUR WAY OUT.**

# TOP FIVE

## WHAT ARE YOUR FAVORITE THINGS TO DO WHEN THE BABY IS NAPPING?

1. _____

2. _____

3. _____

4. _____

5. _____

*Journal:*

**Things I will never do when the baby is napping (*circle all that apply*):**

a) Play the drums

b) Practice Olympic pole vaulting

c) Read William Blake to myself out loud

d) Watch Nick Jr. alone

e) Go for a run when no one is chasing me

f) Make some freshly pressed juice

g) Steam my vagina

h) Go to a swingers party

i) Don't talk to me, I'm sleeping

**If my baby decided to take a six-hour nap tomorrow, I would:** _____

_____

_____.

# PEOPLE YOU MAY WANT TO HAVE AROUND AFTER THE BIRTH

Some people get home from the hospital and want nothing more than to hibernate, preferably for a few months. Even if you seriously do not want to see another adult human being for as long as possible (because seeing one might mean that you have to speak to them or put on a bra), you need to make a few exceptions.

### 1. A Handyman

If shit breaks, nobody in your household is going to fix it. Certainly not you—you have a pineapple-size piranha attached to your nipple—and your partner has very likely gone into total IS THIS MY LIFE NOW?! panic mode (which, in some people, produces a condition not dissimilar to full-body-and-mind paralysis).

Have a handyman on speed dial. Because if your dishwasher or washing machine decides that now is a good time to go on strike and you don't know who to pay to fix it, oh god, you will be sad.

## 2. The FreshDirect Person

While Chinese takeout exists mostly to make women who have just given birth feel better about life, sometimes you need stuff that the Chinese place won't deliver. Like Ben & Jerry's Coffee, Coffee BuzzBuzzBuzz! And beer. And, okay, diapers.

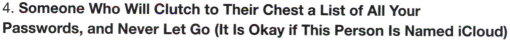

Enter the FreshDirect person, who will climb endless flights of stairs only for the joy of (directly!) depositing the (fresh!) groceries that you requested right there on your kitchen floor. Just be sure to make someone else put them all away—you really shouldn't be lifting things. Right?

## 3. Your Mother/Mother-in-Law

If having your mother/mother-in-law around normally makes you a tad irritable because please stop explaining how to live my life, this might change in the days immediately postpartum. It can be incredibly reassuring to have a seasoned, practiced mom around to tell you that yes, that color poop is normal, and do things like hold the baby while you pee and shower. She may even cover part of the night shift so you can sleep a few hours in a row.

## 4. Someone Who Will Clutch to Their Chest a List of All Your Passwords, and Never Let Go (It Is Okay if This Person Is Named iCloud)

There will come a point each day—hopefully a few of them—when your baby will sleep. Every newborn manual and grandmother in the world will tell you that when the baby sleeps, you need to sleep, too, but if what you want to do is watch *Friday Night Lights* instead, it's a virtual certainty that you will collapse onto the couch, turn on the television, and be greeted by a large, aggressive message that reads:

* Please enter your iTunes/AppleTV/Internet password *

Why? Because God has a sick, sick sense of humor and knows that of all the fucking things on the planet that you can't remember right now, passwords are at the top of the list.

Summary: The first few weeks of a baby's life are a precious time, and a time during which you get to call the shots. Ask for help, accept it when it is offered, and kick out anybody who you don't want around (they'll forgive you, promise).

# GET OUT OF THE GROCERY STORE IN UNDER THREE HOURS

AVOID OLD LADIES WHO THINK YOU'RE DOING IT WRONG! CHOCOLATE! CONFUSING
FORMULA LABELS! MASSIVE BOXES OF DIAPERS! TEARS!

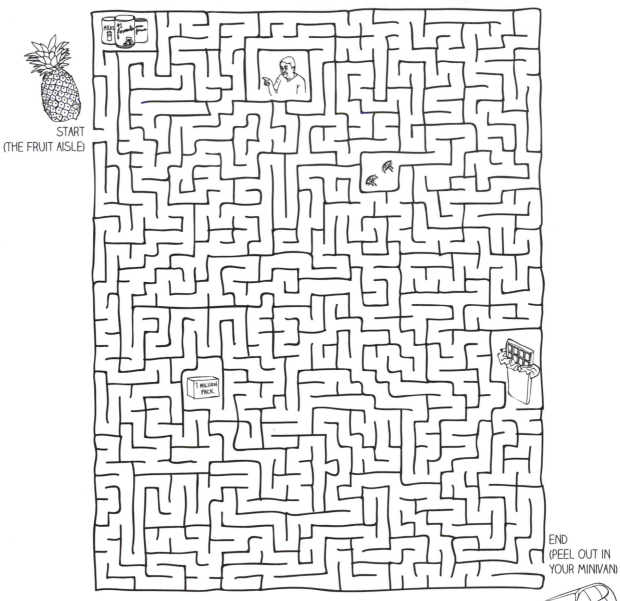

START
(THE FRUIT AISLE)

END
(PEEL OUT IN
YOUR MINIVAN)

# THINGS YOU SAID BEFORE YOU HAD A BABY

**THEN**                                                              **NOW**

| THEN | | NOW |
|---|---|---|
| "Of course I'm going to make my own baby food! What do you need, like, a blender and a bunch of vegetables? People who buy baby food are so lazy." | **DIY** | "Thank you, corporations, for mushing up peas for me so that I do not have to spend my four free minutes of time every day in the company of a blender and eighteen postage-stamp-size Tupperwares." |
| "My child will sleep from 7 p.m. to 7 a.m., just like French children." | **SLEEP** | "…Or not at all, ever." |
| "I will not do 'baby talk,' and certainly not in the presence of other adults." | **TALK** | "I have now started referring to my own bathroom activities as 'going poo-poo.' This is as excellent for my marriage as it sounds." |
| "It's so important to sit down at the table and eat three balanced meals a day." | **MEALS** | "My diet consists of Kudos bars and glasses of wine carefully timed so as not to interfere with a breastfeeding schedule." |
| "My baby will never lick a floor." | **GERMS** | "My baby licks floors professionally. Mostly in places like airports. And this keeps him quiet, so this is fine." |

# DINING, FANCY BABY-STYLE

Baby food has come a long way since the days when you just mushed up some carrots with a fork and called it a day. Nowadays, prepared baby foods include ingredients like "magnesium sourced from a blend of waters" and "organic flavor." What all this health means: Now even parents who make their own baby food get to feel guilty if it doesn't contain essence of holy basil leaf.

Hooray, progress!

*Find the foods listed below, all of which are actual ingredients in actual baby foods being sold in actual stores at this very moment.*

ACAI
ALMA
AMARANTH
BLACK CARROT
   EXTRACT
CRIMINI MUSHROOMS
CURRY LEAVES
EDAMAME
ELDERBERRY JUICE
GROUND CHIA

HEMP SEEDS
HOLY BASIL LEAVES
JAPONICA RICE
KALE
MILLET
PROBIOTICS
QUINOA
SALBA
WILD ALASKAN
   SALMON

S Y J L P Z O G Q Y V I T A F X J I L E A B A L M A J H H N
C H U N V Z U O S L M N C D Q O O N J D Q Z W F C T K K O M
C I G M V Q T Z I I I S A A Q R H V X Q W Q B V T G T E M L P
T D D J K V S W M D N R R S E V A E L Y R R U C Q D L L Y D
O R W Z Y J S Y O F R W T Q E V K C B N Q Q W Y A A Z R B A
I X H E U S Q Z W G X T X F N L K M Q Q E C F Z S J G S A R
B V M M I B K J A F K Z E J S M D I C S E J S N A D F K S H
O J J J K L E C B H T R Q H E P N U P A K H B I R I L
R I R P C Z X N Q X Z Z O H Y V O N R V B K R B X Z S L R
P T O B D V A Q R T Y D R Y A C A H H B S W L B V Q G R L H
U H F E Q W C E G X M O R N D Z W L U A E U D R J R B P E W
O O L Y O S Q H V B I G A H V W N F L F J R H F P D A V
A A Q T O U T K S H L C C P A I M A O Z E U R H C F Y I V W
K I P B O Q D E F U K F K Y M Y D B G G U J E Y C I G G E U
S W H C E A V X Z C H S C M G L F A I L A A N W J V Y C S Z
F E P C D G U X A G X K A D I E U F W P Y P B L E U F P I B
E C J Z D S N H U O K R L W V J P O V F U F L V T I P N W
F D A A D N J B W Z S I B F W P H N S O G P L R A F U C W P
E C A I E X U S K I C R I M I N I M U S H R O O M S I A E A
I D I M F S K O T S E M S J J C W K O E C B D S U R J B V L
M V P D A Q R F R D L D G T A B M E L S X F B K I M C H Q A
O M M Q F M K M S G E J F R G W O U I B N F D R N J J U C E
T R Y L V Z E R Q E J I I D A B X V Y A N D N Z M D I Y O H
H C S N C J Y Z S M F C T E L L I M S W X A Y W L N I O X J
I J Q G U X N P B U E N T H P Y F B H A F V G U O T A H S C
Y T V T M X M D L N L P A M A R A N T H C T M A Q Y C R L S
C K E E C E K F D C U K Y U O S L D I J Y V F A B J A A N E
I L Q V H P Y C N J N C R U V Q Z L Q N W N J J G V F Y Q X
Y U H I O Z T C W F R M I F V V F F H K Z V A V Z C Q X G X
K K U L L I V D L L L Q E W P E R C E G L C I G A Z I S Q L

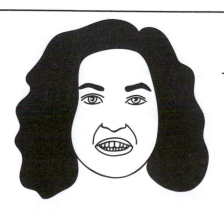

—my baby is on a gluten-free
paleo organic housemade
holy basil diet

ok —

# WEIRD BABY THINGS

*Match the weird baby thing on this page to its description on the opposite page.*

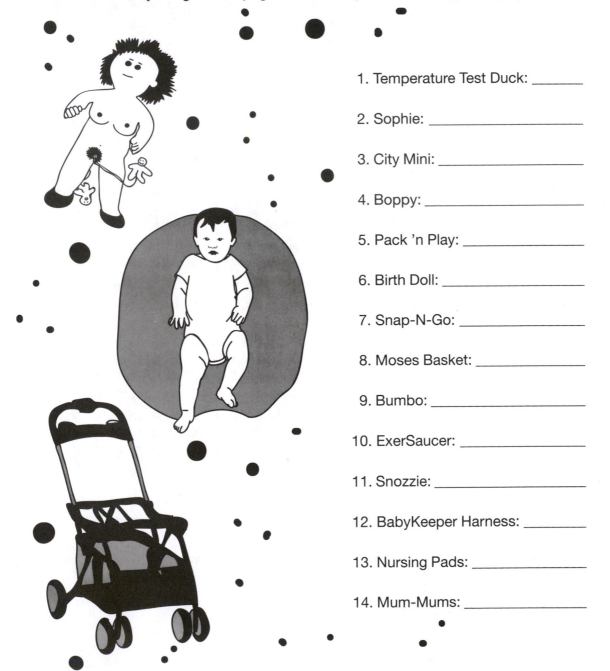

1. Temperature Test Duck: _____

2. Sophie: _____

3. City Mini: _____

4. Boppy: _____

5. Pack 'n Play: _____

6. Birth Doll: _____

7. Snap-N-Go: _____

8. Moses Basket: _____

9. Bumbo: _____

10. ExerSaucer: _____

11. Snozzie: _____

12. BabyKeeper Harness: _____

13. Nursing Pads: _____

14. Mum-Mums: _____

a) Extremely uncool wheely-thing that allows you to transfer your baby from the car to wherever you're going without waking her up, and is therefore the best.

b) Anatomically correct stuffed woman with removable baby and detachable placenta used to visually communicate to small children exactly (like, exactly) how the miracle of childbirth works.

c) Baby cage that requires three fully-grown adults and six trips to the computer to figure out how to assemble.

d) Expensive bed for newborns that your newborn will never sleep in.

e) Ergonomically designed resting area for a nursing baby, aka a pillow that costs extra because it's round.

f) Plastic giraffe that is French and thus chic. At some point, it became mandatory to own at least three. They cost $28 each.

g) Stroller of choice for cool moms who do things like jog.

h) Toy that you place in your baby's bathwater to determine whether it is too hot, presumably because you do not have hands capable of fulfilling this function.

i) Maxi pads for your boobs.

j) Sling that you can hang on the door of a public bathroom so that your baby has somewhere to chill while you pee.

k) Strangely delicious banana-flavored air crackers that you will find crumbs of in your purse for the rest of your life.

l) Very cute, chubby-looking baby seat that your baby will use for approximately two weeks before discovering that he can vault out of it.

m) Donut-shaped party for your baby that keeps her in one place and ecstatically happy for up to two minutes. This is how you do things like bathe and pee.

n) A "bracelet" fashioned from a piece of cloth intended to be used as a tissue when the real thing isn't handy. As a bonus, this product allows you to wear your child's boogers as accessories (now that's love).

# HOW TO MAKE OTHER NEW-MOM FRIENDS

If you haven't made a bunch of new-mom friends by the time the baby arrives, then please allow us to present you with your official Certificate of Being Normal. The secret is that the 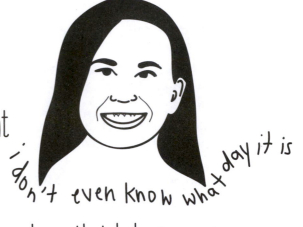 real desperation doesn't set in until you have that baby in your arms, your maternity leave to contend with, and you start needing some allies. As a new parent, you feel every single minute of the day tick by when you're not sleeping, a purple raisin-baby is screaming and flailing in your face, and you're busy doubting every instinct you have. Also, you probably have poop on your face.

Once you get your bearings a little bit and get comfortable with the idea of leaving the house with your babe, it is time to venture out into the world in search of your compatriots.

## 1. Hit Up Storytime at the Library

As soon as your baby is old enough to swim in the germ pool, go to storytime. As you sit cross-legged in a semicircle, awkwardly smiling while trying to remember the words to "Itsy Bitsy Spider," shoot laser beams of quiet desperation through your eyeballs at the other moms. Remember that they are just as sleep-deprived and confused as you are, and that they smell like baby barf, too. Just go talk to them. You have so much in common already!

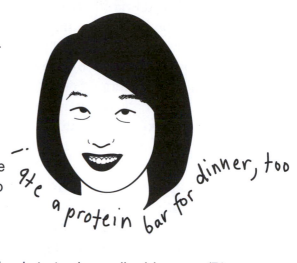

*ate a protein bar for dinner, too*

The proper method of furthering a new-mom relationship without seeming like a potential stalker is to trade email addresses. (Phone numbers are usually exchanged after you've vetted each other via email enough to ensure that you're not handing out your digits to a scary weirdo.) Sign your emails with both your name and your baby's name, to help your new friend keep it straight, and hopefully they'll do the same. Everyone will probably confuse and/or forget one another's names anyway, which is normal when the status quo is accidentally leaving one shoe at home and having a booger stuck to your eyebrow.

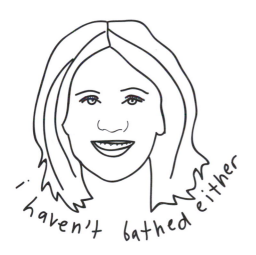

*haven't bathed either*

## 2. Go to Every Free Introductory Class

Baby classes are hilarious, and also ridiculous. There are all kinds of structured activities available for kids these days, and many offer classes for small babies, too. Many of these are outrageously expensive, but most offer the first class for free.

Take, for example, the "baby gym": a class for which you can pay $900 per six-month "term" so that your infant, whose primary concern is making out with the floor, can engage in "structured movement" in close proximity to other infants (who are also making out with the floor). The "teacher," a recent high school graduate, will sing "Mary Had a Little Lamb" with such grand embellishment that she is clearly banking on a member of the Grammy Selection Committee being in attendance. She will lead you through various exercises, alerting you to their "tremendous!" yet also tremendously vague and pseudo-scientific benefits, while your baby tries to escape.

### 3. Reconnect with Old Friends Who Are New Moms

You know all those pretty cool people you lost touch with after high school? Facebook stalk them, and reconnect with the ones who also have kids. Even if they're far away, a digital support network is a big help on the days when you need someone to remind you that you're not doomed to spend eternity in a blazing inferno of hellfire because you let your baby watch fifteen minutes of *Sesame Street* so that you could chug coffee and stare at your Instagram feed in peace.

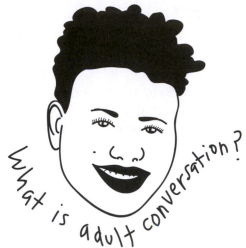

Your new-mom friends will not be your old college friends, the ones who know you inside and out and remember staying up all night with you drinking 99 Bananas liqueur and watching repeats of *Friends* while eating very large bags of bagels. You might have been in a punk band, while your new friend starred in a very good small-town production of *Fiddler on the Roof.* You might be a vegetarian, and she might bake whole pigs in a pit in her backyard. Maybe you're an atheist, and she gives it up to Jesus.

It matters very little whether your new-mom friends truly understand your soul, because they will understand why your boob is hanging out of your shirt and why you haven't showered in three days, and both of those things are more important.

As different as everyone will be in your brand-new, ragtag team of sleep-deprived zombies, the reality is that you need one another. These women will become your closest allies: the ones who will babysit at the last minute because you desperately need help, who will tell you how great you look when your eyeballs are about to fall out of your face, and who won't judge you for feeding your eight-month-old white bread for lunch because that's all he'll eat.

Find your friends. They're out there, and they need you, too.

# YOUR BABY'S #1 HOBBY IS POOPING IN THE TUB

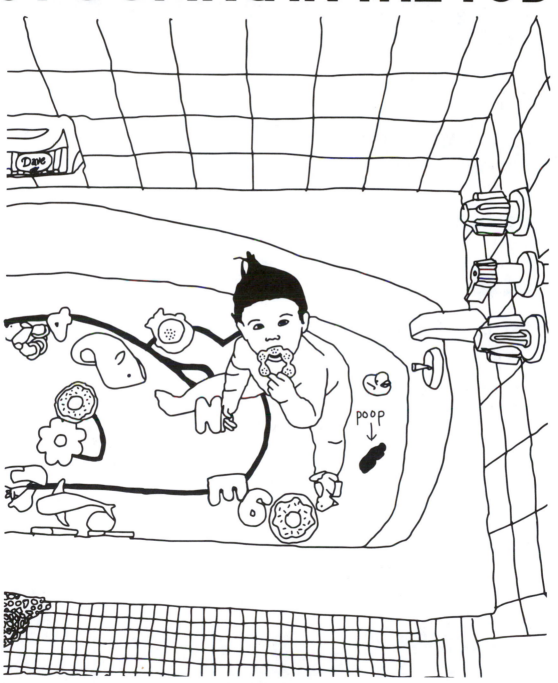

# FROM "BFF" TO "ANOTHER THING YOU NEED TO CLEAN UP AFTER"

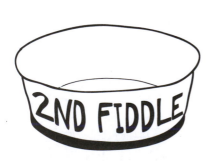

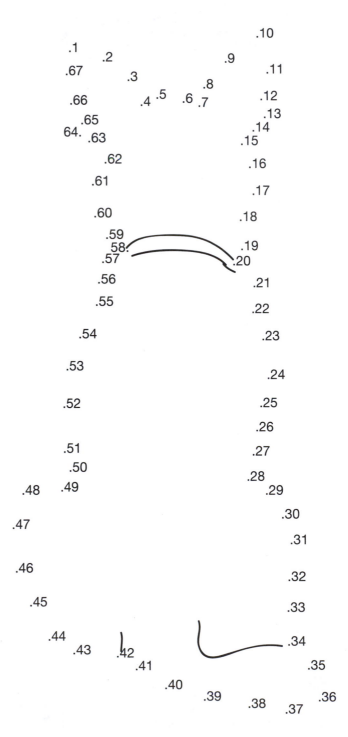

# THINGS IN YOUR HOUSE THAT ARE IN SERIOUS TROUBLE NOW THAT YOU HAVE PROCREATED

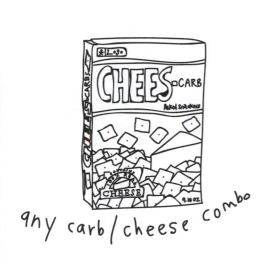

any carb/cheese combo

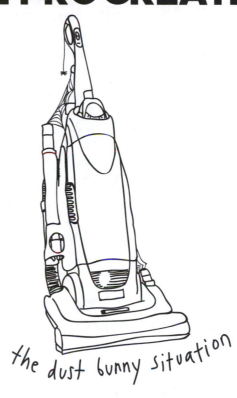

the dust bunny situation

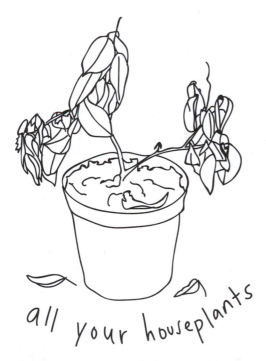

all your houseplants

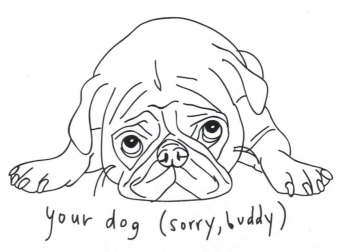

your dog (sorry, buddy)

# COLOR THE SOOTHING MANDALA OF DIAPER BAG ESSENTIALS

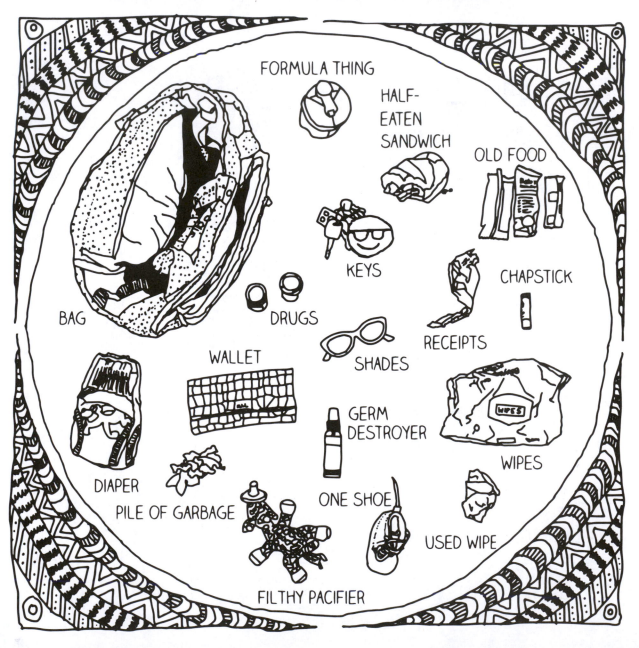

# POSTPARTUM CHECK-IN

As of today, I have officially been a parent for _____ weeks.

My baby is _____ pounds.

I only want to wear _____.

The part/s of my body that is/are annoying me the most is/are my _____.

I really love my _____, though.

If I even think about _____, I want to throw up.

The biggest to-do on my checklist right now is _____.

The best thing that happened this week was _____.

The worst thing that happened this week was _____.

When I think about my partner, the primary word that comes to mind is _____.

I really miss _____.

I'm so excited to _____.

When I hold my baby, the first word that comes to mind is _____.

Mostly I feel pretty _____.

I want to eat _____ RIGHT NOW.

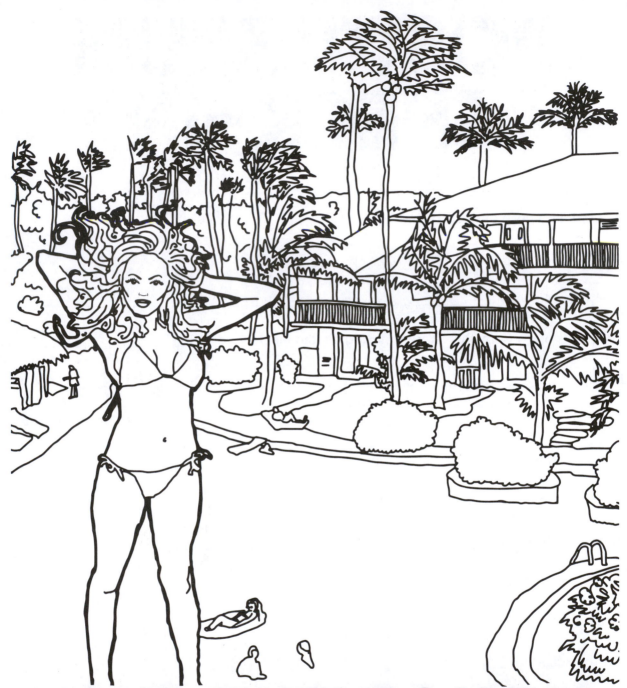

# YOUR FRIENDS WHO DON'T HAVE KIDS

# FIND THE FIVE DIFFERENCES
# BETWEEN THE TOY CABINETS

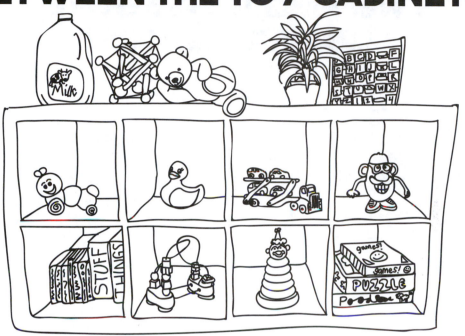

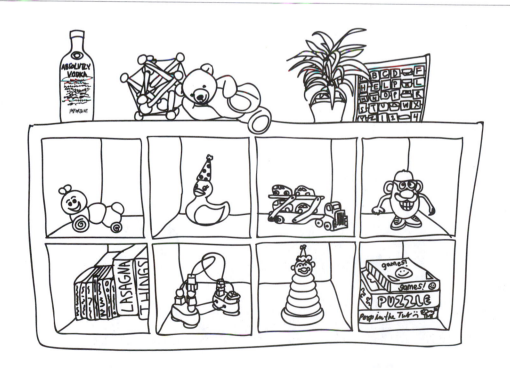

# REMEMBER: IT NEVER HURTS TO DOUBLE-CHECK THAT YOU'RE WEARING PANTS BEFORE LEAVING THE HOUSE

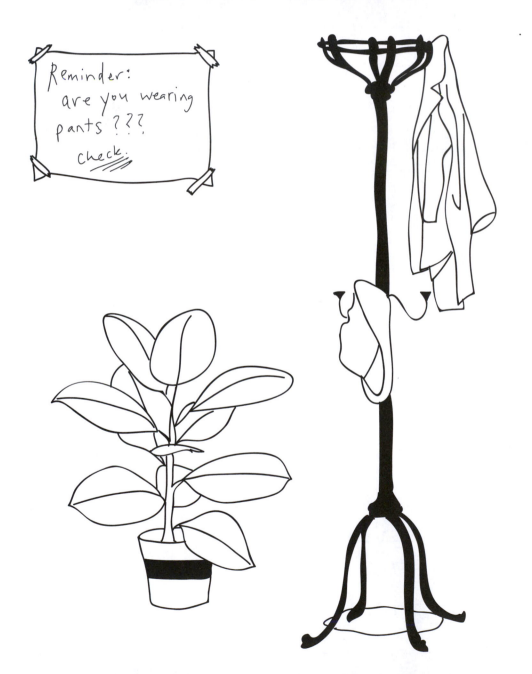

# THE 5 BEST SNACKS TO KEEP HANDY IF YOU'RE BREASTFEEDING (OR JUST HUNGRY)

One thing about breastfeeding is that you will be starving pretty much all the time. Your body is feeding another human being with its big magical boobs! Feed the boobs.

Obviously you will have food in normal places (like, say, the kitchen), but you should also stash it everywhere else, like in your purse and on your nightstand. Getting caught without snacks while breastfeeding is like releasing a fire-breathing dragon into a lush jungle: Shit is gonna burn. Be prepared.

### 1. Crackers
Any kind you like! Your partner will love it when you wake them up in the middle of the night, loudly crunching and spilling crumbs into the sheets. This is a very nice revenge technique for not being the one to birth a person. It also helps with nausea.

### 2. Granola or Protein Bars
These are delicious, there are a million kinds, they keep forever, and you can buy them anywhere. They may also enhance your milk supply if they contain oats. You can buy fancy organic ones if you are still that type of lady. (Just give it nine months; then you will realize that your baby's favorite food is "floor" and start viewing the feeding process for both yourself and your child less as "an opportunity for acquiring a wide range of nutrients" and more as "GET FOOD IN STOMACH.")

### 3. Nuts
Buy a large bag (online, as you will not be going to the store, thank you very much). Dole it out into individual portions—a two-pound bag should be about, what, three servings? Put these giant bags into your purse in case you ever decide to leave the house again.

### 4. Peanut Butter
It comes in individual pouches now, so you can whip one out anywhere and confuse people into thinking you're still pregnant. It also contains fat, fiber, and other things that are supposedly healthy.

### 5. Fruit
If you're into that sort of thing.

# TEXTS YOU MAY SEND YOUR PARTNER WHILE SEVERELY SLEEP-DEPRIVED

Come in bedroom I can't reach remote and if I move baby will wake up 😭 😭

oh my god your mom will NOT STOP HUMMING AND I CANT THINK

Need wifi pw and my mind is doing that thing where it can't do anything help please

Did u walk the dog before u left???? Say yes or I'm giving it away

our child just projectile shit onto the laundry basket 😭 💩 💩 💩 💩

Do you want anything from fresh direct? Look in the ready made meals section. They have wings. Beer??? 😵

My nipple is literally about to fall off can you google if that can happen please??? Would do it myself but if I put her down she yells and also I'm scared 😭

Stop at store and get 2 boxes diapers 5 cans sugarfree red bull one case white wine (cheap) and whatever else you want, but don't spend too much money ok???

The baby has a spot on her back. It might be a freckle but I can't tell. Should I call the pediatrician?

Everything on sex and the city is wrong except the parts with Miranda in them.

When are you coming home because dying. 😭 😭 😭

Come fucking home.

hi

# PRIORITIES

You may have noticed that once that baby arrived, your priorities shifted ohhh, just a touch, and not always in the ways you'd expect. Maybe, for example, it is now super important to make sure your hair looks nice, but you can take or leave interaction with any and all adult members of the population. Remember: Anything is possible while in the throes of postpartum hormones.

*Place each of the words or phrases below into the appropriate column.* (We put "cheese" in the correct one for you.)

My partner, Concealer, Cheese, Adult conversation, Clean sheets, Me time, Mascara, A nice neat bikini line, Anti-wrinkle cream, Cute spit-up cloths, A hairbrush, Cheap spit-up cloths, Pants that fit, The Boppy, Cooking, The Bachelor, Chinese food delivery, Name-brand diapers, On Demand, Wine, A co-sleeper, Baby mittens, Advice, Protein bars, My friends, Giant maxi pads/adult diapers, Leaving the house, Tylenol, Clean dishes, Help, A really good book, Nursing pads, Instagram, Baby-wearing, US Weekly, A cool-looking stroller, A clean kitchen, A clean car, Showers, Any liquid, Antibacterial wipes, My mother-in-law, A white-noise machine, My mother, Physical contact with my partner, This activity book

# THINGS I CAN'T LIVE WITHOUT

*Cheese*

# THINGS I DON'T GIVE TWO SHITS ABOUT

# Quiz

## ARE YOU A GOOD MOM?

It's something we all wonder from time to time (also known as "every day, and constantly").

*Find out once and for all how you're doing with this whole "parenting" thing.*

1. How many times (today) has your child consumed animal hair?
    a) Oh my god, I would freak out—that has never happened, and it never will
    b) I'm pretty sure the answer is "none," but don't hold me to that
    c) At least three. Maybe five
    d) Hair (feline, canine, and/or human) was today's primary food group. On the plus side, I don't need to vacuum anymore

2. What is your child's toy situation like?
    a) I spent our entire tax refund at Buy Buy Baby
    b) Mostly hand-me-downs, plus a few new things
    c) Whatever my mom gave me
    d) An empty toilet paper roll and a box of Kleenex

3. How many hours a night does your baby sleep?
    a) From 7 p.m. to 7 a.m., because my baby is a genius
    b) About eight hours, with occasional wake-ups for a bottle or a diaper change
    c) Significantly less than I would like her to
    d) …Children are supposed to sleep at night?

4. Have you started having sex with your partner again?
    a) Right at the six-week mark! I couldn't wait!
    b) We've done it once or twice
    c) We're in talks. Maybe in a year. Or five
    d) Fuck no

5. What does your baby wear on an average day?
    a) Clean, seasonally appropriate clothing
    b) Seasonally appropriate clothing
    c) Clean clothing
    d) Clothing, sometimes

6. What did you feed your baby?
    a) Breast milk from my boobs
    b) Breast milk from a bottle
    c) Formula
    d) I am exhausted, and this quiz has too many questions

Now tally up your score.

How many As? _____
How many Bs? _____
How many Cs? _____
How many Ds? _____

Flip this page to find out if you're a good mother.

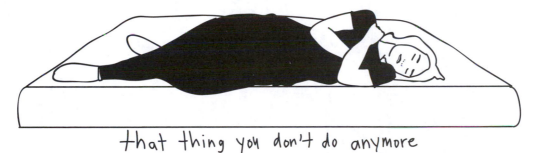

that thing you don't do anymore

Mostly As? Congratulations. You are a great mother.
Mostly Bs? Congratulations. You are a great mother.
Mostly Cs? Congratulations. You are a great mother.
Mostly Ds? Congratulations. You are a great mother.

answers

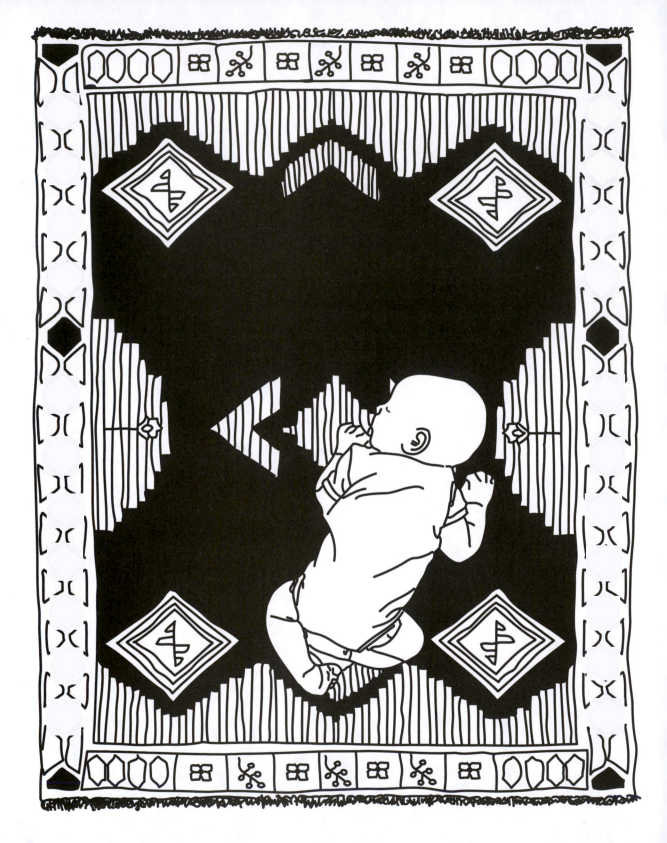

# I'D MOVE MOUNTAINS FOR YOU,

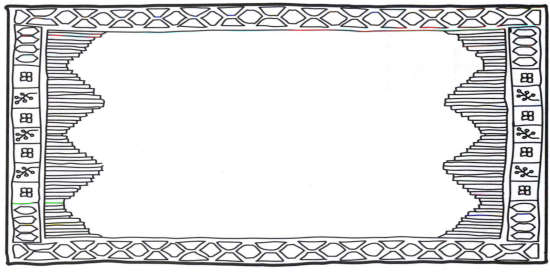

your baby's name here ♡

# dear _____,

You are here at last.

You are (*circle all that apply*):
- a) Extremely small
- b) So beautiful
- c) Already brilliant, obviously
- d) Exhausting
- e) A complete and utter terror
- f) Very, very loud
- g) Preternaturally quiet
- h) Super cute
- i) Such a weirdo

Your favorite things to do are:
- a) Sleep
- b) Not sleep
- c) Cry
- d) Look at my face
- e) Nurse
- f) Make smiley faces that I think mean "I am pooping now"
- g) Poop, generally
- h) Destroy my nipples
- i) Hold on to things (like my hair) with a death grip
- j) Stare at light fixtures like they're Bruce Willis movies

Here are three things that I really, really want you to know:

1. _____

_____.

2. _____

_____.

3. _____

_____.

I'm new at this "mom" thing, but I'm already sure that _____

_____. And I don't know much

about you yet, either, but I already know that you are _____

_____.

Before I get back to:
- a) Feeding you
- b) Hopping up and down like a crazy person
- c) Pumping milk
- d) Trying to figure out how to get you to fall asleep

I want to tell you this: _____

_____

_____

_____

_____

_____

_____.

Welcome to the world, kid. It's a pretty cool place.

love,
    mom

# Acknowledgments

Our biggest thanks to Nina Shield and the crack team at Penguin Random House (especially David Rosenthal, Aileen Boyle, Marian Brown, Alie Coolidge, Kayleigh George, Justin Thrift, Norina Frabotta, LeeAnn Pemberton, and Dora Mak) for allowing us to curse so much in a book about pregnancy. Thanks also to Deborah Schneider and the team at Gelfman Schneider.

Jordan: Erin, you are equal parts brave and weird, and that is a phenomenal combination. Becca Capozzi, Victoria Sanders, Reesa Lake, Karen Robinovitz, Raina Penchansky, and the rest of the crazy-good DBA team: I feel lucky every day to get to work with you. Morgan, Erin C., Elise, Alisa, Mollie: There are no women I'd rather be in the trenches with. Francesca: Thanks for letting me collapse on your floor when I need to. Kendrick: Let's do this "in love" thing forever and ever, okay? And finally, to River and Shea: All that stuff we wrote about in this book ended with your beginning . . . and I can't wait to see where you go. I love you—both of you— the most.

Erin: Jordan, your enthusiasm is otherworldly and contagious—thank you for being the best business and writing partner a person could have. Thanks to my ragtag crew of mom friends for always reminding me that none of us really knows what we're doing: Emily Levy, Sue Gilpin, Kate Novotny, and Sarah McGroarty. Joan Fortin, Jerome Williams, George Williams—I'd love you even if you weren't family. Thanks to Colin Fitzpatrick and Julian Smyth for letting me get weird. Cait Weiss: I'll be reading your book next. My biggest thanks is to Kyle, my partner in this life and all other realms—I love you. To my dear Lucy Williams: I love you impossibly. This, like all things, is for you.